THE
EASY DOES IT YOGA
TRAINER'S GUIDE

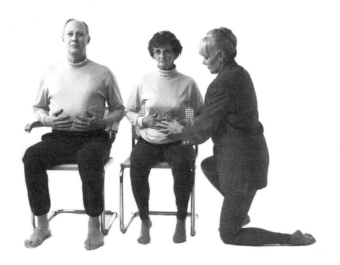

Alice Christensen

Founder, American Yoga Association

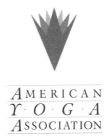

AMERICAN
Y·O·G·A
ASSOCIATION

KENDALL/HUNT PUBLISHING COMPANY
4050 Westmark Drive   Dubuque, Iowa 52002

Inquiries should be addressed to:

The American Yoga Association
513 South Orange Avenue
Sarasota, Florida 34236
(813) 953-5859
(800) 226-5859

Executive Editor for the
American Yoga Association: Patricia Rockwood
Photographs by Herbert Ascherman, Jr.
Design by Linda Gajevski
Technical assistance by Hunter Chisholm

Copyright © 1995 The American Yoga Association

All rights reserved. No part of this publication may
be reproduced, stored in a retrieval system, or trans-
mitted, in any form or by any means, electronic,
mechanical, photocopying, recording, or otherwise,
without the prior written permission of the copyright owner.

ISBN 0-7872-1190-7

First Edition

Printed in the United States of America
10   9   8   7   6   5   4   3   2   1

CONTENTS

PREFACE

Easy Does It Yoga has been my "pet project" ever since the day I walked into a new Yoga class in the late 1960s and found the students to be all seniors! This class challenged my creativity in adapting the classical Yoga exercises so that everyone could enjoy and benefit from the class. I learned a lot from these enthusiastic students.

My parents had retired to Florida by then. When I visited them and saw the needs of retired people firsthand, I realized that there was — and is — no training in the United States for growing older happily and staying healthy and independent. We would have long talks about my parents' fears of being put into a nursing home. I developed this book for them and for all of us who are growing older in our country, with the knowledge that the great potential of wisdom, experience, and beauty in older Americans everywhere can be protected and encouraged by this program, which helps maintain independence in later years. This will be a valuable asset to them and to our country. I am very proud to offer this revised edition of our trainer's guide, which will enable anyone to help a relative, a friend, or a client learn these simple techniques for better health. I dedicate this book to my mother and father, Harry and Clara Harvey, with great respect for their courageous lives.

The production of this book would not have been possible without the generous donations of time and energy made by so many of our staff, students, and friends here at the American Yoga Association. First, my deep gratitude goes to Stephenson Grant, who organized so many research projects on Easy Does It Yoga and helped me write the first edition of this book. I would like to thank Linda Gajevski and Hunter Chisholm, who spent long hours designing a beautiful and easy-to-use book. Our models for the photographs were Mladen Golubic, Corrine Goodman, Margaret Pepple, Joy Walworth, and Ed Wardwell; I thank them all heartily for their cheerfulness and patience during long photography sessions. I would also like to thank Cynthia Ingalls, Pattie Cerar, Carol Goodwin, and Carole Guerin for their generous and enthusiastic performance of myriad tasks essential to this work and the work of the American Yoga Association.

Finally, none of this work would have been possible without the support of my two great teachers, Swami Rama of Haridwar and Swami Lakshmanjoo of Kashmir. They were shining examples of the great treasure of one's older years; their older years were the most productive years of their lives. They had trained their whole young lives to prepare for it — and it showed. Even after the age of 80, Lakshmanjoo was a brilliant example of how one ages with dignity and power, and Rama's example of compassionate help with so many people in this world in his older years stands like an inspiration before me and all of us at the American Yoga Association.

Alice Christensen
Sarasota, Florida
March, 1995

INTRODUCTION

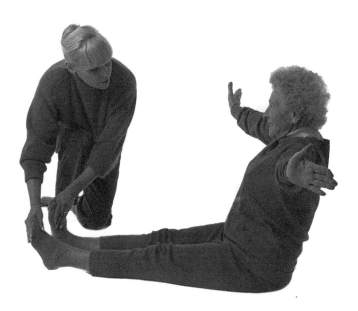

Welcome to Easy Does It Yoga

Congratulations on your aspiration to learn how to teach Easy Does It Yoga. Your contribution to the health and well-being of older adults in your community can make a real difference to your students and to our country. As our population of people over 60 grows to a new, incredible high in the next few decades, Easy Does It Yoga (EDY) can help make the later years happier, healthier, and more fulfilling for our country's older adults.

Easy Does It Yoga was developed by Alice Christensen, founder and executive director of the American Yoga Association, in the late 1960s. She was surprised when she arrived to begin teaching a new class one day and found the room full of seniors, and was touched when one of them remarked, "We didn't tell you we were all grandparents because we were afraid you wouldn't come." Easy Does It Yoga began with this group of older adults and developed into a program applicable to anyone with physical limitations due to age, illness, disability, drug abuse, or simply years of inactivity.

What Is Easy Does It Yoga?

Surveys have shown that Americans of all ages consider the years between 60 and 70 to be the least desirable time of their lives. Those under 65 seem to hold a deep prejudice against the aged, and evidence from many sources reveals that many of us react to old age with fear and dread. Older people themselves, even though they may feel good about their own health, tend to exaggerate the problems of poor health, loneliness, poverty, and loss of independence for other older people.

Easy Does It Yoga is a holistic program of exercise, breathing, and relaxation techniques designed to improve or maintain the health of older people who may be suffering due to chronic disease or multiple functional disabilities. It is also an effective *preventive* program: Practiced regularly, Easy Does It Yoga can help prevent the development of many of the health and functional problems commonly associated with aging, and greatly reduce the likelihood of a person's being forced into a nursing home in later years. The program is most effective when presented as self-administered procedures which become the student's responsibility to implement following an initial training period. Our experience indicates that Easy Does It Yoga is an ideal, low-cost approach that provides exciting new ways of dealing with the problems resulting from retirement, inactivity, and poor health, and provides new life enjoyment for the later years.

The goal of the training program outlined in this book is twofold: to facilitate the training of older people in Easy Does It Yoga techniques to improve their fitness, health, and independence, and to outline motivational techniques that help older people to incorporate the Easy Does It Yoga techniques into their daily lives. Whether you are a therapist, home caregiver, exercise instructor, health professional, or simply someone who wishes to help a parent or friend become stronger and healthier, you will find many useful techniques in this book. Your role is to communicate the correct Easy Does It Yoga procedures adapted for individual needs in such a way that they can be easily learned by your older students, and to motivate and provide a supportive atmosphere so that the techniques will become a part of their daily activity. Your students depend on you to teach them the procedures and for the impetus to practice; to a great extent, from then on the responsibility is in their hands. With your help, your students can learn to help themselves be more fit, independent, healthy, and happy about this time in their lives.

Who Are Your Students?

This program is suitable for many different populations. In this book we use the following definitions: "Frail" refers to those who require some type of assistance in daily living and therefore do not live independently; they may live in a nursing home, a senior residence with daily home care, an ACLF, or at home with round-the-clock care. They may be bedridden or confined to a wheelchair. "Active" refers to those who are able to care for themselves adequately and therefore live independently; while not engaging in vigorous exercise, they are able to walk short distances, drive, or otherwise lead a relatively functional life. Easy Does It Yoga can also be very helpful for those of any age who have been inactive for quite some time due to illness, injury, or substance abuse, and who need to move gradually back to their previous level of activity. In

this case, Easy Does It Yoga serves to gently build muscle tone and strength, as well as instill positive changes in attitude, while the person recovers fully. In the technique chapters, special symbols will alert you to techniques that can be done in bed, a wheelchair, or the pool (see p. 15).

The techniques in this book are suitable for use with either groups or individuals. We highly recommend that you use this book in conjunction with our student's manual, *Easy Does It Yoga for Older People*, which is written in a style especially designed to be interesting and motivating for older people (see Resources, p. 105).

Overview

Chapter 1, "Starting an Easy Does It Yoga Program," suggests how to motivate older adults, how to set up a class, and how to approach various medical problems that commonly appear in older people. Chapter 2, "How to Teach Easy Does It Yoga," presents the most important EDY concepts to keep in mind as you begin preparation for teaching, plus some hints for becoming a more effective teacher. Easy Does It Yoga is different from other exercise programs, and its effectiveness depends upon following the guidelines presented in this chapter.

In Chapters 3 to 7, you will be given step-by-step instructions on how to teach the exercise, breathing, and relaxation techniques of Easy Does It Yoga, along with the benefits of each technique and variations for more or less able participants. The techniques are presented in order of increasing difficulty.

Chapter 8, "Suggested Curriculum Outlines," combines the techniques into several curriculum formats and tells you how to adjust the formats for different populations or circumstances. In the Appendices, you will find a list of all the techniques grouped according to their physical or emotional benefits; an annotated list of additional resources from the American Yoga Association, including information about Easy Does It Yoga training opportunities; and a summary of research to date on Easy Does It Yoga.

We wish you the best of success in Easy Does It Yoga. Please write to us if you have any questions about what you are doing; we would also love to hear about

CHAPTER 1

STARTING AN EASY DOES IT YOGA PROGRAM

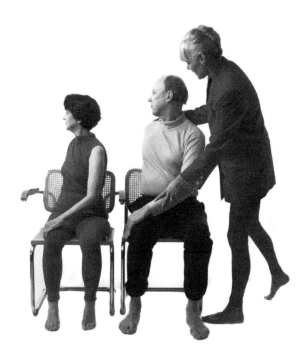

SELECTING PARTICIPANTS

If you are a home caregiver, or a therapist working with an older person individually, set up a time to meet with your student on a regular basis. Frail students will benefit most from more frequent, shorter classes: 20- to 30-minute sessions, five times a week, would be ideal to start. Keep to your schedule as much as possible, and encourage your student to practice alone on the days when you are not there. Your goal is to motivate your student to practice a little every day: Regular practice does a great deal to relieve depression, which will, in turn, contribute to greater well-being and the motivation to continue practicing.

If you are a teacher of Yoga or exercise, or an activities director in a senior facility, you will probably already have the machinery in place to organize a group class. If not, following are some suggestions:

1. Add Easy Does It Yoga to ongoing group or individual sessions.

2. Begin Easy Does It Yoga with students referred to you (either group or individual) by other staff.

3. Introduce several (3-5) students to Easy Does It Yoga individually, then combine them into a group.

4. Enlist volunteers, either individually or from a group meeting.

If you are new to teaching, an encouraging way to start is to begin by training students who are most likely to be successfully rehabilitated and then returned to the community. This type of student is more likely to become motivated, and also less disabled, and thereby easier to teach. With experience, you can sharpen your skills for attempting to work with poorly motivated and more disabled students in the future. Another important point to remember is that students you have worked with who enjoy the program can be valuable assistants and models when working with others and can serve an extremely useful role by helping to organize prac-

9

tice sessions as a part of daily activities in the center or residence. Word of mouth is extremely effective advertising, and a few enthusiastic, successfully trained students can result in many more people who are excited about getting into the program. Frail students especially enjoy working with another student as a teaching helper.

Another effective approach is to train several students in some of the techniques, and then schedule a demonstration program during a group meeting, such as a meal, using the students as models. (See Chapter 8 for a suggested outline of a demonstration program.) If you are enthusiastic and communicate the benefits of the program, and the models demonstrate how enjoyable and easy the exercises are, a significant number of people will be inspired to sign up for a structured program. Encourage students to bring a parent or friend to the program to learn how to train them in Easy Does It Yoga. Anyone, with practice and the help of this training guide, can learn to teach someone Easy Does It Yoga techniques.

SETTING UP YOUR CLASS

First, learn all you can about your students: Find out about any medical problems and try to be aware of their daily schedules. Select a time for your meeting that is at least two hours after meals to allow adequate time for digestion. Suggest to students that they also avoid caffeine for at least an hour before class. The best time of day is one that is free for the students every day, so that they can practice on their own at the same time on days when there is no class.

Meet with your students in a quiet room, preferably one with a door that can be closed. Minimizing distractions in the classroom allows for more concentration as well as better comprehension and subsequent recall of the techniques. If you are teaching in a senior center or residence, ask staff to turn off any intercoms to the classroom, and post a "Do not disturb" note on the door. Students need to feel protected.

Remind students to wear loose, comfortable clothing to class; tight waistbands or girdles will inhibit proper breathing and free movement of the body. Students should wear long pants instead of shorts in order to keep the legs warm, and should bring a sweater or shawl to class to wear for the relaxation period. Encourage students to practice Easy Does It Yoga without shoes in order to exercise the foot and ankle muscles and improve balance; you should teach without shoes as well. It might be necessary to remind certain students to urinate before exercising to prevent incontinence. If any students are in wheelchairs, be sure the chairs are locked in place. For ambulatory students, have a sturdy, straight chair for each; make sure the chairs will not roll or slide easily. A carpeted room is best for students who are learning to get on the floor. You might also try to have some foam mats handy for more comfort, and a few pillows to place under the knees for resting lying down.

FREQUENCY OF CLASSES

Active students in group classes will benefit from meeting one to three times a week, with reminders to practice at home on other days.

Frail students may need daily reinforcement at first. If you are able to provide a daily class, it should be held every day at the same time, in the same place. However, care must be taken to avoid creating overdependence on the instructor. Stress from the very beginning that the students are ultimately going to be responsible for continuing the program. What you need is a balanced relationship of learning and support that is not too distant on the one hand, and not too dependent on the other. Participants who learn the exercises quickly can often be slowly weaned to self-governed practice after only five to ten classes with you. The weaning process consists in both monitoring, as opposed to leading, the exercises during class, and in reducing the number of formal classes per week with a clear agreement with students that they must perform their exercise routine on days when there is no class. Stronger students may be used as a support for training more frail students.

For a group of about five frail students, a possible schedule of teaching might look like this:

Weeks 1 & 2: five classes per week
Weeks 3 & 4: three classes per week
Weeks 5–12: two classes per week

Our experience indicates that within 12 weeks, or 20 to 25 contact hours, virtually all older people, except those with serious cognitive impairment, can learn the basic Easy Does It Yoga curriculum.

Medical Problems

It is up to you to ensure that you know what limitations your students' problems place on their ability to exercise. If you have any doubts or questions, check with the appropriate staff or ask students' permission to speak with their physician. The safety record of the American Yoga Association staff is perfect, and our own staff training and caution are the reasons behind our record. Be cautious!

It is very important that you get your students to talk to you about their problems, as you compare what they say with their records. If you see that students lack understanding of their condition, be careful that you do not encourage them to experiment and practice on their own too soon. Talk to your students, making them aware of how to work around their problems safely and responsibly.

Functional disability due to arthritis, hypertension, stroke, heart disease, chronic obstructive lung disease, constipation, obesity, depression, and anxiety are some of the more common problems that older people face (as do those in any type of rehabilitation program). As well, significant numbers of older people are blind, deaf, paralyzed, or single or multiple amputees. Any successful exercise program must take these problems into account, be adaptable to those problems that cannot be changed, and be cautiously applied to those problems that show promise of responding to rehabilitation efforts. Many of the exercise descriptions in Chapters 3 to 5 are marked by a "caution" symbol to alert you to specific conditions that might be affected by that exercise. Following are some specific suggestions to help you meet the medical challenges posed by your students.

Nonambulatory

Throughout this guide you will see special symbols indicating which exercises may be done in bed (see page 15). For obvious reasons, bedridden students should be worked with one on one. Students in wheelchairs may do most of the seated exercises in Chapter 3, especially if they can be moved to a sturdy chair. Some may even be able to stand for short periods of exercise using a walker or chair for support.

Arthritis and Osteoporosis

These diseases decrease joint function, but exercising correctly frequently moderates pain and stiffness. Because of the brittle nature of arthritic tissue — and this applies equally to limbs affected by osteoporosis — *all exercise should be performed by the student, and the instructor should never attempt to "help" a movement.* On the other hand, physical touching is a very important way to build trust and to motivate the student toward consistent practice. The instructor must find the line between a too-cautious, hands-off approach and an overzealous pushing beyond safe limits. The student with arthritis must be constantly reminded not to exceed the range of motion that can be performed comfortably. No pain and no strain are the key words that should be constantly on your lips.

Hypertension

This disease, frequently associated with hardening of the arteries, is usually controlled by medication. The Easy Does It Yoga exercise program has shown promise as a valuable adjunct to reduce blood pressure (see research summaries in Appendix C), and those with mild hypertension should be encouraged to participate, but with caution and constant monitoring. Pacing is particularly important; be careful to proceed slowly, taking full advantage of every rest and relaxation pause. Those with severe hypertension must be careful to avoid extreme movements of the head, neck, shoulders, and arms, and also should approach the inverted (head-down) exercises with many gentle warm-up trials. In some cases, several months of practice may be needed to perform the exercise completely. A slow pace, no extreme movements of the upper body, and slowly working into the inverted poses are the important points to remember. The breathing techniques are particularly important, because those with hypertension often breathe shallowly.

11

Depression

Depression can be as crippling as arthritis, by decreasing one's engagement in the "outer world," limiting appetite, and curtailing social activities. We have observed many instances where depressed moods have lifted after only one or two weeks of Easy Does It Yoga. In our work with older people, we have noticed a close relationship between depression, inactivity, and poor breathing habits. The Easy Does It Yoga program reestablishes regular activity and improves breathing, as well as having a direct effect on improving enjoyment of life.

Chronic Obstructive Lung Disease

The incidence of emphysema, bronchitis, asthma, and other lung diseases seems to be on the increase. The Easy Does It Yoga program deals with these problems by teaching better breathing habits, improved posture, increased flexibility of the chest wall, and greater strength of the respiratory muscles. Pace the program very slowly and ensure that the Belly Breath is learned well. We do not recommend exhaling through tightly pursed lips, a technique to prevent early airway closure, preferring instead to improve muscular control to slow and deepen exhalation. Within this general context, you will have to evaluate each older person individually to recommend the most appropriate breathing technique.

Deafness and Blindness

Hearing or vision loss should never exclude a person from Easy Does It Yoga classes. The teacher's demonstrations for each exercise, as well as the copy and diagrams in the *Easy Does It Yoga* student's manual, permit those with hearing loss to participate, and clear, unmistakable spoken commands, and hands-on guiding of movements, allow the visually impaired to gain the benefits of exercise, breathing, and relaxation procedures. When helping blind students to learn, remember that the student must be active and that your role is only as a guide; you should not force any movements. Always tell a blind student what you are going to do (e.g., "I'm going to put my hands on your shoulders to help you turn") so that he or she is not startled by being touched without warning.

Strokes and Heart Disease

The effectiveness of exercise for stroke victims varies depending on the location and severity of brain damage. Creative solutions to each person's particular disabilities are the responsibility of each instructor. Those afflicted by heart disease are limited primarily by needing a slow pace, and students with pacemakers should not try to raise their arms above shoulder height.

Anxiety

Everyone suffers from mild anxiety from time to time, but chronic anxiety takes a tremendous toll on the body, draining energy resources and keeping the body in a constant state of stress. In older persons, the effects of anxiety can be magnified when the body is not exercised: tension in the muscles builds, breathing remains constricted most of the time, and the mind has no rest from the whirling thoughts and feelings that feed the anxiety. The best Easy Does It Yoga techniques for students dealing with chronic anxiety are the breathing and relaxation exercises.

Back and Neck Problems

Back problems are very common among adults: Some estimates say that over 20% of adults have some chronic back pain. Among older adults, back pain may be enhanced by a lifetime of poor posture, weak back and stomach muscles, or chronic degenerative disks, especially in the lower back and the cervical spine. Most exercises in the Easy Does It Yoga program will not make a back problem worse, but you will need to approach all bending movements slowly and carefully, individualizing the exercises for each student as needed. Many students may be afraid of exercising for fear of injury. Don't insist; instead, show how the exercises can be simplified so that students can feel that they aren't helpless with a back problem; that there is always something they can do to slowly build their strength. Reinforce the idea that inactivity causes even worse problems. Over time, they will experience how regular exercise results in strength, flexibility, better posture, and fewer muscle spasms. Daily practice of Easy Does It Yoga will also help to prevent injury by strengthening ankles and hips to reduce the likelihood of falling and by strengthening back and stomach muscles, improving steadiness and balance.

Chronic Pain

When chronic pain is due to arthritis or other joint problems, inactivity often makes the pain worse. In this case, moderate exercise is often recommended to reduce stiffness, strengthen muscles, and reduce the incidence of spasms. Pain also causes a great deal of stress, and Easy Does It Yoga is ideal for helping students learn to cope. Exercise stimulates the production of endorphins in the brain, reducing pain sensations and increasing feelings of well-being and calmness. Relaxation techniques can also be very helpful in reducing pain. The novelty of the Easy Does It Yoga program often functions as a temporary distraction that breaks the constant expectation of pain. On an acute level, some students have told us that they have experienced success in using breathing and relaxation techniques to reduce discomfort when undergoing medical or dental procedures.

Incontinence

Often seen as an inevitable result of aging, incontinence can be corrected with a specific muscle-strengthening exercise in addition to the regular Easy Does It Yoga routine. This technique is described in the chapter on floor exercises.

Obesity

Affecting an ever-increasing percentage of our population, obesity is sometimes regarded as an obstacle to exercise and is often blamed for limited movement that is actually caused by tight ligaments and stiff joints. Obese participants should be careful not to overstretch connective tissue, and particular attention is usually needed to maintain motivation to keep them active in the program. The joints of the hips, knees, and ankles seem to be more vulnerable to injury in obese people, and care should be taken accordingly.

Paralysis and Amputees

As with deaf and blind students, these problems challenge the creativity of the instructor to adapt the specific techniques to the abilities of the individual student. Neither paralysis nor loss of limb makes Easy Does It Yoga impractical or impossible. In addition to the effects of even a modifed exercise program, Easy Does It Yoga can offer a great mental change in outlook for these students.

Recent Surgery

While most health professionals recommend resuming normal activity as soon as possible after a surgical procedure, it is important to take special care with exercise. Your students should obtain written permission from their physician before resuming their exercise routine after surgery, though they should be encouraged to do the breathing and relaxation techniques often during their recovery period to help cope with anxiety and discomfort.

Nutritional Impacts

A poor diet can cause symptoms such as depression, fatigue, irritability, and weakness. Too much caffeine, for instance, can cause the same symptoms as acute anxiety. A student who is malnourished or who eats improperly will have trouble concentrating and may even feel faint or fall asleep during relaxation and breathing exercises. While Easy Does It Yoga is best practiced about two hours after eating, be sure students have had some nourishment prior to coming to class. A section in the student's manual discusses some important nutritional concepts for older people. Read and discuss these ideas with your students. Some important points to bring up are how to minimize sugar and fat in the diet, how to get enough protein, fiber, calcium, and other nutrients, substitutes for caffeine and alcohol, and sensible snacks. If you can, have wholesome snacks such as fruit juice and whole-grain crackers available in class.

CHAPTER 2

HOW TO TEACH
EASY DOES IT YOGA

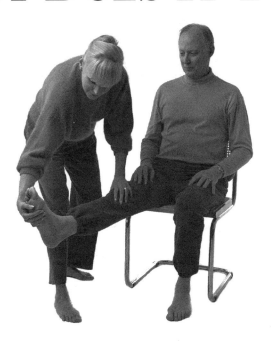

In this chapter you will learn some fundamental principles for teaching adapted Yoga techniques. Yoga is different from traditional forms of exercise, and it's important to follow the directions explicitly.

In Chapters 3 to 5, the exercises are presented in increasing order of relative difficulty, making it easier to see how the techniques can be used for people with varying capabilities, and how you can gradually add more difficult exercises as your students become more confident. Many exercises have variations for more or less active students.

The following symbols are used throughout the technique chapters to refer to techniques that may be used for special populations or environments:

    may be done in bed

    may be done in a wheelchair

    may be done in the pool

For students in wheelchairs, be sure the chair is in a locked position and that feet are firmly supported. Most seated exercises are marked with the bed symbol; these may be done sitting up on the side of the bed, but make sure feet are firmly supported on the floor. Many warm-up exercises, such as the Shoulder Roll, may be done lying on one's side, exercising one arm at a time. Almost all floor exercises can be done in bed lying down. Seated exercises may be done in the pool sitting on the steps; standing exercises should be done holding on to the edge of the pool for support.

EASY DOES IT YOGA TEACHING CONCEPTS

Always Breathe through the Nose

The importance of breathing in and out through the nose cannot be stressed enough. Most students are unused to exercises in which breathing is such an

15

important aspect, so they need to be reminded with each instruction. Breathing through the nose affects the nervous system differently. It also improves concentration and eyesight. Some participants, especially those with severe obstructive lung disease, may have to exhale through tightly pursed lips for a while to keep airways open, though this should be seen as a temporary measure if at all possible. Some students ask if they should be breathing as deeply during the exercises as they do when they are practicing the Belly Breath or Complete Breath alone. Because of the body's movements during exercise, it will not be possible to practice the exact Complete Breath sequence while exercising, but students should be encouraged to breathe as deeply and completely as they can at all times.

Counteract Negative Thoughts with the Positive Opposite Idea

Always emphasize the potential for growth and achievement in your students. If, for instance, a student is unable to raise her or his arm in an exercise due to shoulder stiffness, say: "I know your shoulder will definitely get stronger and more flexible" and offer a simpler variation to achieve that objective. You should always stress to students that success in Easy Does It Yoga does not mean perfection in the performance of exercises, but rather the greater awareness of one's body and mind.

Another way you can reinforce this concept is to look for objective signs of improvement and tell your students what you've observed. It is a common phenomenon in Easy Does It Yoga for students to believe that progress is not being made because change happens slowly. You as the instructor will begin to notice changes such as brighter complexions, more strength, greater range of motion, better posture, and less depression. Many times these exercises even improve students' appearance due to better grooming and more attractive coordination of clothing. Look for these things and don't fail to mention them.

Use Caution When Introducing New Movements

The ability to adjust rapidly to new demands diminishes with age, so add new procedures to the repertoire slowly — especially in the first few weeks of class while you are still getting to know your students and their particular physical conditions. Be sure that you know what medical problems your group is facing and how the Easy Does It Yoga techniques will affect them so that no injuries will occur. It is particularly important to be aware of arthritis, pulmonary, and cardiovascular problems.

When teaching the exercises, be extremely alert and observant for signs of pain and circulatory or respiratory difficulty. Stress over and over again: "Do not strain; the exercises should not cause you pain. Exercise slowly, gently, and in a relaxed manner." If your students follow these directions, the possibility for any complications is extremely remote, but every deviation slightly increases risk. It is your responsibility to ensure that your directions are clear enough for your students to follow them explicitly. We would even suggest that if you cannot trust a particular student to perform the procedures correctly, you should consider making arrangements for a few private sessions. In class, stand next to this person and use him or her as a class model, which will reinforce correct practice.

MOTIVATING OLDER PEOPLE

The goal of Easy Does It Yoga is twofold: teaching safe and effective techniques that are designed to improve fitness, health, and independence, and motivating older people to perform the techniques on their own as an integral part of their daily activities. This section summarizes some of the important attitudes that will help you motivate students to practice on their own.

Treat Older People as Adults

Frequently, management of groups of older people leads to an authoritarian control that strips older people of responsibility for basic life requirements. In the Easy Does It Yoga program, as much as is possible, older people are to be treated as the mature and responsible individuals they are; this often results in more self-initiated behavior.

Respect Older People as They Are Now

Many older people, especially the frail elderly, have experienced a gradual erosion of responsibility for work, family, and community life, and suffer from low self-esteem due to the feeling of not being needed. To counteract this tendency, constantly communicate during the sessions that what they are doing and experiencing at this moment is important to you and others in the group. Getting older people to talk about their present-moment experiences reduces the risk of loss of reality orientation into past or future fantasies. Students become happier and proud to contribute to the class.

Use Humor

Easy Does It Yoga exercises must be presented as noncompetitive with the abilities and progress of others as well as with one's own self-imposed expectations. With the multiple functional losses that most older people undergo, combatting their common feelings of failure needs a warm, lighthearted, and fun environment. Easy Does It Yoga techniques must be presented as enjoyable to do if they are to be self-administered after the initial learning period. Don't be shy about relating your own experiences to illustrate some point in class. Treat your students as your friends.

Use Direct, Clear, and Nonthreatening Communication Skills

Speak in a loud, clear, and low-range voice. Avoid simplistic language; older people may move more slowly, but their brains are as sharp as ever. To avoid losing the attention of those with hearing difficulties, place those students in the front of the class, closest to you, and talk from in front of your group or student, making eye contact. Frequently ask if students can hear you.

Do not "loom over" older people in chairs; try instead to use a chair yourself, or even kneel or squat beside them.

Use the pronouns "I" and "you" rather than "we" as in, "How are you feeling today?" or "Now I'd like you to raise your arm" rather than "How are we feeling today?" and "Now we're going to raise our arms." This establishes a connection between you and the student so you are clearly talking to them rather than at them.

Easy Does It exercises should be presented as "win-win" experiences. In other words, there is no wrong way to do any exercise. If a particular movement seems complicated and difficult to learn, break it up into simpler segments.

Use Caution

Be alert to the reduced adaptability of older people, watching for dizziness, hyperventilation, or signals of pain. Many times we have instructed particular older people to not do certain exercises, or to use only a modified procedure, always emphasizing that this is only a temporary measure and communicating the full expectation that with practice, the disability will improve and normal procedures can be adopted. Be especially watchful when the participant is visibly tense while exercising, when anyone is coming up from an inverted or supine position, and after the relaxation exercise. Be sure every student has a sweater or shawl to wrap up in during the relaxation to avoid becoming chilled; the covering also helps people feel protected during that quiet time (see Chapter 7).

Talk About Practical Physical Benefits

Most older people have not exercised regularly in the previous 30 to 40 years, and the presentation of specific physical benefits is a powerful motivating tool. Learning to relax and get rid of tension, and discovering more limberness, greater strength, and less irritability are extremely satisfying experiences that you can use to constantly reinforce exercise behavior. Certain physical effects are universally reported and can be used as motivators also. Especially common are reduced musculoskeletal pain, reduced sensations of numbness and tingling, and fewer problems with twitching muscles in the face, neck, and shoulder areas. Helping your clients find ways that the program has benefitted them is extremely valuable both for their own motivation and for that of other members of your class. Make it a point to mention the benefits of each exercise every time it is taught in the first few weeks of class, and ask your students to talk to you about what is happening to them in class and at home; take several minutes of class time for this.

Be Supportive and Enthusiastic

We have unfailingly noted the beneficial effects of a positive and enthusiastic approach that also includes physically touching the student. Many older people live alone; add that to our culture's strictures against physical touching, and the result is people who are often lonely for human contact. A hand on your student's shoulder once in a while, or gently guiding them into a particular position, will usually be much appreciated. Naturally, never force a student's body into position; simply guide the student to move or stretch in the proper way. Don't be shy about communicating your caring and enthusiasm; at the same time, be aware of your students' "personal space" and respect their individual preferences. As a group leader, your attitude will set the mood of the class.

Help Your Students to Generalize the Exercises

Easy Does It Yoga techniques can be done during many daily activities such as watching TV, playing cards, or waiting in line. Make notes to yourself of how the exercises can be incorporated into daily activities, and discuss these with your students at every session. Ask students to supply examples of how they have practiced their techniques at home between sessions. Find out which activities your students enjoy most, and help them think of ways to work Easy Does It Yoga into those activities.

Individualize Your Students' Timetables

Avoid failures as much as possible by adapting movement goals to the limitations imposed by physical conditions. This will be easier in a class composed of people at similar levels of ability. In any class, however, there will always be people of different strengths. Teach while standing next to the weakest ones — without making it obvious that you are doing so.

USING THE INSTRUCTION SECTION

Each of the techniques in Chapters 3 through 7 is presented in four sections:

How Will This Exercise Help?

A brief list of some of the more important physical benefits of the exercise is provided. This material is an important motivational tool, and you should present these to your students in practical terms. For example, when teaching the Shoulder Roll, which improves the range of motion of the shoulder joint, you could say something like this: "The Shoulder Roll will loosen your shoulder joints and make it easier to reach above your head." Repeat the benefits often during class, and encourage your students to tell you how the exercises have helped them.

Instructors Should Remember . . .

This section includes important tips on correct movement and pace that are not made clear by the verbal instructions. This section also alerts you to any cautions for specific medical problems that may be affected by the technique.

Verbal Instructions

A brief script is presented with each exercise to show you the correct teaching procedure. Even if you are an experienced teacher, use this script at first to be sure you are including all important information for safety and effectiveness of the exercise.

Variations

This section offers suggestions for how to vary the exercise for either more or less able participants.

INSTRUCTOR PREPARATIONS

Learning the Exercises

In order to effectively teach a technique, you must know how it feels to practice it yourself. Pay particular attention to which muscles are used, and what types of strain the exercise puts on particular joints and systems. Learn the breathing patterns that are used for each exercise so you have them memorized and can instruct smoothly without having to refer to notes during each exercise.

In our training seminars we often provide heavy gloves, knee braces, blindfolds, and other "props" to help teachers understand how it feels to have arthritis, joint problems, cataracts, and so on. Try it yourself and see how it feels to exercise with limited movement. If you know what problems your group has, practice as if you had those same problems.

Hints for Becoming a Better Teacher

As with any new skill, teaching a class requires preparation and practice. If you have never taught exercise before, we suggest that you practice teaching several techniques to your parents, grandparents, or friends before plunging into a class situation. Ask for honest feedback about your presentation. Be sure you are confident of the details of each technique before you teach it to actual students. Another excellent way to prepare is to practice teaching in front of a mirror.

As an instructor, you are demanding more of your body and mind than usual. Protect yourself from "burnout" by practicing some simple preventive measures:

Take care of yourself. Get in the habit of doing some exercise and relaxation daily. Eat sensibly. Get enough rest. Your students will look to you as a model of someone following a healthy lifestyle, and you should not ask them to do anything you are not doing yourself.

Don't overload yourself by teaching more than you can comfortably manage. A beginning trainer should start with one or two classes per week for several months (or if working with individual clients — one or two at a time). Recognize your personal energy levels and don't exceed them. Learn to recognize your body's stress signals and practice appropriate techniques to reduce harmful reactions.

Be clear about your role. Remember that Easy Does It Yoga is not a cure-all, and you cannot possibly solve everyone's problems. Your role as a trainer is to teach techniques that help people help themselves, not to take on the problems of all of your students. Learn the resources available in your institution or community for psychological, financial, medical, social, legal, and other help — and use them.

Questions to Ask to Check on Students' Progress

Easy Does It Yoga increases students' self-esteem by improving daily functioning, increasing independence, and improving health and well-being. Constantly ask your students about how they are feeling, and point out any changes you see in their appearance, carriage, complexion, temperament, and ability. Following are some questions to ask to get students to think about how they are changing as a result of their regular exercise:

How's your stamina? Can you walk longer distances? How about climbing stairs? Are you feeling stronger? Is it easier for you to get out of your chair? Can you turn your head a little further than before? Is it easier to shop? To drive?

How about regularity? Have any of you noticed that your constipation is better? How are your knees (shoulders; ankles; legs; arms; hip joints)? How's your arthritis? Blood pressure? Has your doctor commented on your health and strength? Are your eyes brighter?

What activities can you do more easily now than before you started exercising? Do you find that some things are more fun to do now? Do you feel more alive? More alert? More interested in things? How's your energy level? Is it easier to get out of bed in the morning? Is it easier to get to sleep at night?

Has anyone given you a compliment this week? Are family and friends telling you how wonderful you look? Do you find yourself more outgoing than before? How about liking people better? Feeling that others like you even more? Are you more interested in new activities and getting out more than before? Are you feeling more on top of things? Are you less crabby and irritable?

Are you less short of breath? Do you find yourself doing the deeper breathing automatically? Can you sing better? Is it easier for you to get dressed? Button your clothes? Zip up? Tie your shoes? Put on your stockings? Is it easier to reach up to wash or brush your hair? Can you take care of your house or apartment better? How's your balance? Can you get down on the floor and back up more easily? Are you able to reach to a higher shelf for something you need?

Suggestions For Class Discussions

Discussions in class add variety, stimulate thought, and help to reinforce the idea of total fitness by extending the idea of health into other aspects of life. Some ideas follow:

Common Sense and Safety. This is probably the most important topic, and you should talk about this often in the first few weeks. Many people, in their excitement over the good feeling that they get from doing the techniques, may overdo, resulting in strain and disappointment. Stress "easy does it," going at your own pace, starting slowly. There is no competition in Easy Does It Yoga; everyone benefits from the techniques, no matter how far one can stretch or bend.

Self-Esteem and Body Awareness. Talk about the idea of making friends with your body. Most of us see only the parts of our physical body that we do not like; how about concentrating instead on the things we do like? How about giving our bodies credit for all they have done for us over the years? A body that is appreciated works better! (See broader discussion of "Body Talk" on p. 22.)

Anytime Poses. Students are encouraged to practice the Easy Does It Yoga techniques at odd times of the day, to reinforce their usefulness in various situations. Draw out examples such as practicing breathing exercises while waiting in the doctor's office, leg exercises while watching TV, and balance exercises while talking on the telephone.

Good Nutrition. Be aware of good eating habits and talk about, for example: what constitutes a good breakfast; nutritious snacks; how to get enough calcium; how to cut down on salt, sugar, fat, caffeine, and alcohol; and how to shop wisely for food. Use the *Easy Does It Yoga* student's manual for ideas, and supplement with information from your own reading.

WHAT EVERY CLASS SHOULD INCLUDE

Chapter 8 will give you some suggested curricula to help you organize your classes. Following are two important sequences that should be a part of every class. Practice these sequences so that you can lead them smoothly without referring to notes.

The Warm-up Sequence

Do this sequence at the beginning of each class session as a way for students to gently start moving and become aware of how their bodies are feeling today.

The exercises in this sequence are small movements to be done gently and slowly, almost like a series of stretches after one has been asleep for a while. As you demonstrate the exercises, make your movements slow and at half capacity and your students will mimic your attitude. Encourage students to practice this warm-up sequence any time of day they feel like giving their bodies a stretch. All these movements can be done by wheelchair clients.

Verbal Instructions

1. **Sit up straight in your chair, arms at your sides. How does your body feel today? This simple sequence will help you find out. As you do these exercises, observe your body and try to notice how your body responds. If you notice some stiffness or soreness in some of your joints or muscles, you should remember to take special care of those areas as you go on to more active exercises.**

2. **Start by lifting your shoulders, one at a time, up toward your ear, then down. Repeat a couple of times on each side.**

3. **Slowly lower your chin toward your chest. Then lift it up so you are looking up toward the ceiling (but don't let your head fall back). Then slowly lower your head again and repeat. Next, gently tilt your head to the left, then back up and tilt to the right. Repeat. Now turn your head gently around so you are looking over your right shoulder, then turn and look over the left. Repeat.**

4. With hands on your knees, slump forward, tucking your chin. Breathe out. Now breathe in and arch your back in the other direction, pushing your chest forward. Repeat, breathing deeply but gently through your nose.

5. Raise your right arm over your head and bend it toward the left. Lean toward the left and slowly reach down toward the floor with your left hand, leaning your body to the left and tilting your head left as well. Don't strain. Now straighten, lower your right arm, and repeat on the other side.

6. Starting with arms at your sides, lift your right arm up in front, then up over your head or as far as you can reach comfortably. Make a fist and push up toward the ceiling. Then lower your right arm and lift the left arm. Repeat, stretching a little further if you are experiencing no discomfort.

7. Stretch your right leg out in front, and straighten it. Now lift it an inch or two off the floor. Rest your heel on the floor and pull your toes back toward your face. Relax. Pull back again, two more times. Then rotate your ankle in both directions, about four times each way. Repeat with your left leg.

8. Wrap your right arm around under your left, and then wrap the left over the right. Take a deep breath and then squeeze your breath out as you give yourself a good hug. Repeat with right arm on top.

Rest Sequence

The Rest Sequence focuses attention on mind and body. It gives the student a structured experience of relaxation that can be done whenever it is needed for a calming, refreshing effect.

Use this sequence after every three or four exercises, or any time you feel students may be straining or becoming fatigued. Note that this is not a replacement for the complete relaxation technique done at the end of class, but simply a periodic rest. After the first instruction to relax completely, the pause should be about one minute. It is important to talk through each of the three complete inhalations and exhalations, then let students relax completely for one minute with no talking.

Verbal Instructions

1. Here's a great relaxation and rest sequence that you can use any time you need it to relax and refresh.

2. Sit way back in your chair with your hands in your lap. Close your eyes.

3. Let your body relax completely. Be as limp as a rag doll. [Pause one minute.]

4. Take a deep breath through your nose, breathing in completely; then breathe all the way out through your nose.

5. Breathe in again and fill up; breathe out and relax.

6. Focus on your breath as you breathe in again, filling up, then breathe out, letting your whole body relax.

7. Just breathe normally and rest now. [Pause one minute.]

8. Now gently take a breath and stretch as you open your eyes.

"Body Talk"

Many older students have poor self-esteem, often stemming from feelings of dislike of and disconnection from their bodies. In every class, you have an opportunity to help students improve their relationship with their physical bodies by instilling appreciation and respect and by learning to become more aware of how the body feels and what it needs. Use the following discussion to understand this concept and pass it on to your students.

Many people approach exercise with the idea that they are going to "whip into shape." This is contrary to one of the most important concepts in EDY practice — nonviolence. In our classes, we introduce the idea of acknowledging the needs and "feelings" of your body as if you were considering the needs and feelings of a good friend. You probably would not demand that a friend strain past his or her physical limits — yet how often do we push our body to the point of strain, pain, or exhaustion? You probably would not insist that a friend go to work when ill, yet how often do we keep working when our body is crying out for rest and recuperation? You probably would not insult your friends by criticizing their figure or face, or pointing out signs of age, yet how many of us stand in front of mirrors every day and disparage our own looks and shape!

To be really successful in Easy Does It Yoga you must be able to achieve a balance between necessary change and acceptance of what is. You need the desire to set and attain physical goals and improve your appearance so that you look your best, with confident posture and a healthy glow; but also you need an appreciation of and pride in your own best qualities as well as the acceptance of your limitations without self-blame or shame.

An Exercise to Build Better Communication with Your Body. If you could hear your body "talk" to you, what would it say? What kinds of feelings might your body express? When was the last time you really listened to your body's needs and feelings? Have a conversation with your body right now. Get into a comfortable seated position, close your eyes, and think about the relationship you've had in the past with your body throughout your life; then think about the relationship you have now. Now quiet your mind and relax. Start your conversation by greeting your body; imagine you are standing in front of a mirror and your body is talking to you. What does it say? How does it look? Take ten minutes or so and record your conversation with your body.

Have you noticed how few people can accept a compliment gracefully without denying it, downplaying it, becoming embarrassed, or changing the subject quickly? When was the last time you gave yourself a compliment? Isn't it about time?

22

CHAPTER 3

CHAIR EXERCISES

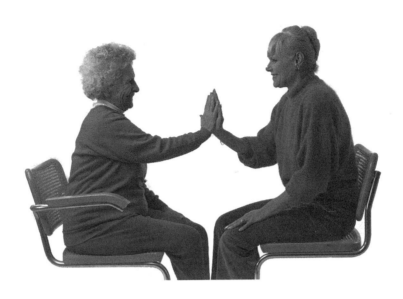

This section begins with some simple movements designed to warm up the body's nervous and circulatory systems. These exercises (pages 24 through 31) can also be done standing, for more active groups.

Rest frequently (see Rest Sequence, p. 21) — at least after every three or four exercises. Frail students will need to rest more often. It is important to remember that people need instruction in how to rest; most people do not relax completely unless taught step by step. You can also build in rest times by inserting brief discussions about the exercises, what benefits your students have noticed (see page 19 for ideas on questions to ask), or any other health-related topic that may arise.

In the "Verbal Instructions" section, instructions in brackets are notes to the trainer. You will see, for instance, instructions to "repeat twice more" or "repeat on the opposite side." Understand this to mean that you should go back to Step 2 and repeat the verbal instructions as your students perform the exercise. It's important, especially with frail students, to talk them through each step of each exer-

cise to be sure they are breathing and moving correctly. Other instructions in brackets will tell you to "count to three" as students hold a position. Count out loud, and pace your count according to your students' abilities. More active students can hold for a longer count; frail students will need a quicker count at first. The idea is to make it a habit to include some period of holding each position, no matter how briefly.

Frequently ask students for feedback about how a particular movement felt. This will encourage them to pay more attention to their bodies as well as help them avoid strain by learning to become more aware of how their body feels at all times.

When introducing an exercise that requires a forward bend, stand close to your student to provide support if needed. If you have more than a few students in class at one time, stand near the student who is most frail, or have students practice one at a time so you can offer support to each one.

See curriculum outlines in Chapter 8 for suggestions on how to combine techniques sequentially.

ARM REACH

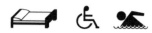

How Will This Exercise Help?

Maintains and improves the range of motion of the shoulder joint, upper spine, and ribs. Strengthens the arm muscles and stretches the muscles of the ribs and torso. Improves ability to reach above shoulder level. Helps to loosen the chest wall and strengthen some respiratory muscles, which improves breathing.

Instructors Should Remember . . .

Those with exceptionally stiff or sore shoulders should not strain or cause pain by lifting too high. Keep arms stiff. Remind students to breathe in *and* out through the nose.

 Pacemaker, shoulder joint problems, severe hypertension.

Verbal Instructions

1. **Sit up straight, with your arms loose at your sides. Breathe in and out three times through your nose, deeply.**

2. **Now, slowly breathe in as you raise both arms in wide circles to the sides and up toward the ceiling. Remember to breathe through your nose. Look up.**

3. **Make fists and hold your breath as you push your fists up toward the ceiling. Keep arms straight. Hold.**

   [Count to three.]

4. **Now breathe out as you lower your arms. Relax. How did that feel?**

   [Repeat twice more.]

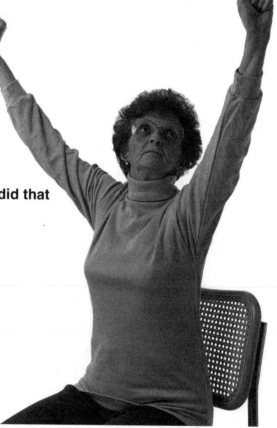

Variations

For very frail students, begin by lifting one arm at a time, using the same breathing pattern: Breathe in as you lift the arm; hold as you push the fist up and count to three. Relax.

Students who cannot lift their arms above their head should lift as high as they can and still push out from the body.

ELBOW ROLL

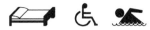

How Will This Exercise Help?

Maintains and improves the range of motion of the shoulder joint and strengthens the muscles of the shoulders and upper arms. Helps to loosen the chest wall and strengthen the respiratory muscles, thereby improving breathing.

This exercise is important for the ability to raise the arms, a movement essential for grooming, eating, dressing, and other daily activities.

Instructors Should Remember . . .

All movements must be made very slowly, with continuous emphasis on never going to any extreme or causing pain. If hands cannot reach top of shoulders, place on chest as high as possible without strain. Elbows should move in large, smooth circles.

 Shoulder joint problems, severe hypertension.

Verbal Instructions

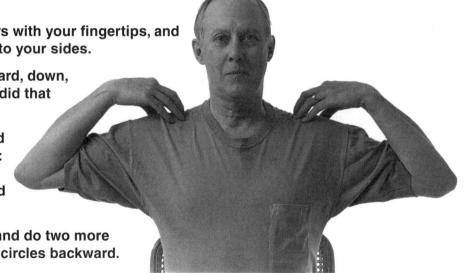

1. Sit up straight in your chair. Breathe normally throughout this exercise.

2. Touch the top of your shoulders with your fingertips, and raise your elbows straight out to your sides.

3. Slowly circle your elbows forward, down, back, and then up. Relax. How did that feel?

4. Lift elbows out to the sides and circle in the opposite direction: backward first, then down, forward, and up. Relax. How did that feel?

5. Lift elbows to the sides again and do two more circles forward, then two more circles backward.

6. Rest and relax. Breathe normally.

Variations

Begin with a simple warm-up: Rotate the elbows in small circles with hands on the chest.

Another variation that stretches the rib cage: Bring elbows together in front of the body, breathing out, and stretch them back horizontally as if they could touch in the back, breathing in. Repeat three times.

SHOULDER ROLL

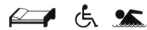

How Will This Exercise Help?

Improves range of motion of shoulders, upper back and ribs. Strengthens muscles of the shoulders, upper torso, and arms. This movement is vital for the free use of the arms in self-care activities such as eating, grooming, reaching, and driving a car. Also valuable for the relief of muscular tension in the upper back which may be causing pain.

Instructors Should Remember . . .

Emphasize slow, controlled movements that extend, flex, elevate, and depress the shoulders as fully as possible, and avoid painful, extreme movements.

The hands can rest in the lap, or the arms may hang loosely at the sides. After learning the movements, the shoulders should roll in continuous and smooth circles, with the head stationary.

⊖ Shoulder problems, severe hypertension.

Verbal Instructions

1. Sit up straight in your chair and let your arms and shoulders relax. Breathe in and out three times through your nose.

2. Lift your right shoulder, letting your arm hang loose at your side or rest in your lap. Now roll your shoulder forward, down, gently back, and up in a circular motion. Relax. How did that feel?

   [Repeat for a total of three circles forward with the right shoulder.]

3. Relax and shake out your right arm. Breathe normally.

4. Now raise your left shoulder and roll it forward, down, gently back, and up. Relax. How did that feel?

   [Repeat for a total of three circles forward with left shoulder.]

5. Relax and shake out your left arm.

6. Now lift your right shoulder again and this time roll it backward first, then down, then forward, then up in a circular motion.

7. Relax. How did that feel?

   [Repeat twice more, then do three backward circles with the left shoulder.]

8. Relax and rest.

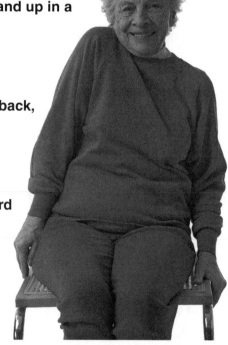

VARIATION
DOUBLE SHOULDER ROLL

Verbal Instructions

1. Sit up straight in your chair. Let your arms hang loosely at your sides or in your lap.

2. Lift both shoulders, roll them forward, down, gently back, and up. Continue in a smooth circle for a total of three circles.

3. Rest and relax.

4. Lift your shoulders again and roll them in the opposite direction: Backward first, then down, forward, and up, in a smooth motion for a total of three circles.

Variations

After mastering the above techniques, your students may perform the exercise after tightening all the arm muscles and making fists.

THROAT TIGHTENER

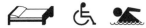

How Will This Exercise Help?

Increases circulation to the head. Improves self-confidence and helps lift moodiness. Stretches and tones the muscles in the neck and throat, helping to remove wrinkles from the throat.

Instructors Should Remember . . .

Repeat to each side, alternating. Students with disk problems in their neck should be careful not to strain.

 Shoulder problems, severe hypertension.

Verbal Instructions

1. Sit up straight, hands on your hips.

2. Take a deep breath in, through your nose. Hold your breath and thrust your chin gently forward, stretching the muscles of your throat.

3. Now breathe out through your nose and relax back.

    [Repeat, thrusting chin to the right, then relax. Repeat to the left. Do a total of three thrusts in each of the three directions.]

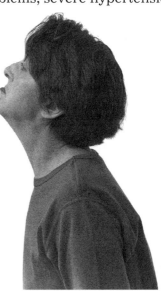

ARM CIRCLES

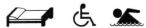

How Will This Exercise Help?

Limbers the shoulder joints, and strengthens shoulder and upper back muscles, facilitating activities such as reaching overhead, carrying, and other everyday movements. Keeping the arms stretched tight with palms up strengthens and tightens upper arms.

Instructors Should Remember . . .

Students with arthritis or bursitis in their shoulder joints should use caution; start with smaller movements.

 Shoulder problems, severe hypertension.

Verbal Instructions

1. Sit up straight in your chair with feet flat and arms at your sides. Breathe in and out three times, through your nose.

2. Stretch your arms out to the sides at shoulder height. Push your palms outward, fingers together, as if stopping traffic on either side of you.

3. Breathing normally, through your nose, slowly rotate your arms in a large circle forward, rotating your arm as far around as you can. Do 5 slow circles.

4. Relax. How did that feel?

   [Repeat, rotating backward this time.]

Variations

Students with shoulder joint problems may begin with smaller circles, but the same outstretched position, palms outward, should be maintained.

ARM SWING

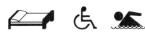

How Will This Exercise Help?

Expands the rib cage, increases vital capacity and circulation, and is invigorating and energizing. Helps relieve breathing problems and depression.

Instructors Should Remember . . .

Be sure students have enough room so that arms can extend straight sideways without running into a neighbor. Remind students to breathe in and out through the nose.

Verbal Instructions

1. Sit forward in your chair.

2. Stretch your arms straight ahead, level with your shoulders, and breathe out. [A]

3. Now start to breathe in deeply and push chest and stomach forward as you open your arms wide to the sides and back as far as you can behind you without straining. [B]

4. Now breathe out as you slouch forward again, and bring your palms together in front of you.

5. Continue the motion, breathing in as you stretch your arms out and to the back, straightening your back; and breathing out as you slouch forward and bring your palms together.

6. Rest and relax.

   [Repeat three to five times.]

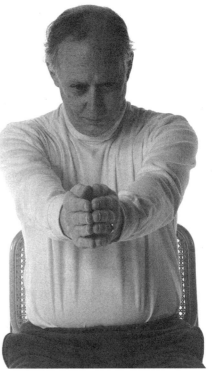

A

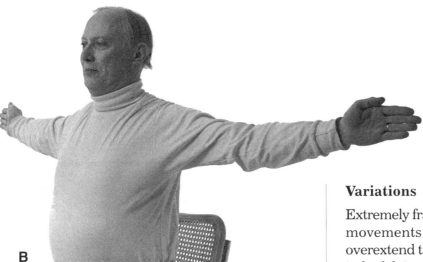

B

Variations

Extremely frail students should start with only small movements forward and back, and should not overextend the back. This exercise can also be done in bed, lying on one's side, with one arm at a time, working up to three repetitions on each side.

NECK STRETCHES

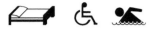

How Will This Exercise Help?

Maintains and increases the range of motion of the joints in the neck and cervical spine. Gently stretches and strengthens the muscles at the sides and back of the neck.

This exercise is important for the maintenance of head rotation, a movement needed hundreds of times daily, and for the reduction of tension-induced pain in the upper back and neck by the relaxation of tension. One is unable to drive a car safely with a stiff neck; this exercise improves the ability to look behind when driving and at other times.

Instructors Should Remember . . .

The neck is very vulnerable to extreme, jerky, and forced movements. Emphasize slow, gentle movements, bending the neck only until the opposing muscles pull tight, and never bending the neck backward. Only the head, not the shoulders, should be moved. Ask students if they feel any dizziness, racing pulse, or pain. Students with disk problems in the neck should do only the variation where the head is gently turned from side to side.

It's important to stress that the shoulders should remain relaxed at all times; many students tend to lift their shoulders toward their ears. Constantly remind students to "relax your shoulders." Note that the hands are to be held on the neck at all times; this forms a supportive "collar" that will help prevent injury to the neck.

⊖ Cervical spine problems, severe hypertension.

Verbal Instructions

1. Sit up straight in your chair. Breathe normally throughout this exercise.

2. Gently bend your head down and to the right without bending your upper back, so your chin comes down toward your collarbone while looking to the right as far as you can. Put your left hand up to the left side of your neck to feel the muscles stretching. Hold for a few seconds, breathing normally.

3. Now bring your head back up straight and bend down and toward the left. Push your chin down toward your collarbone while looking to the left as far as you can. Put your right hand on the right side of your neck and feel the muscles stretching tight.

4. Relax. Massage your neck with both hands [see page 32].

5. Next, keeping your hands on your neck, gently tilt your head to the left, bring it back up straight and tilt down toward the right. [Repeat twice more.]

6. **Still keeping your hands on your neck, look straight ahead and slowly turn your head to look over your left shoulder. Slowly turn back and all the way over to the right shoulder.** [Repeat twice more.]

7. **If these movements feel fine, try a gentle rotation: Slowly lower your right ear toward your right shoulder, next drop your chin toward your chest, then gently bring your left ear toward your left shoulder, and slowly bring your head up straight. Relax. How did that feel?**

8. **Repeat the rotation in the opposite direction: Slowly lower your left ear toward your left shoulder, next drop your chin toward your chest, then gently bring your right ear toward your right shoulder, and slowly bring your head up straight. Relax. How did that feel?**

Variations

For students with cervical disk problems, or who complain of neck pain (or for very frail students), do only very slight movements of the turning variation (Step 6) and be sure that the neck is supported at all times with both hands.

MASSAGE

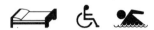

How Will This Exercise Help?

Helps remove stiffness in the joints and muscles and improves circulation, making exercise easier and more pleasant, and reducing the possibility of strain or injury. Helps put students in touch with their physical bodies, which leads to greater self-esteem.

Instructors Should Remember . . .

The point of this exercise is not to press hard with the hands and fingers (which many older adults have difficulty doing) but simply to increase warmth in the affected area. Students should be instructed to use their whole hand when rubbing a joint, not just the fingers. Each joint should be massaged for at least 30 seconds. Encourage students to massage their joints several times during their exercise class as well as at other times during the day.

Verbal Instructions

1. **To massage your shoulders: Start by supporting your right elbow in your left hand. With your right hand, gently rub your left shoulder, using your whole hand — not just the fingers [A]. Rub the entire joint for about 30 seconds. Don't press hard with your fingers; the point is to warm up the joint with your palm, not to "dig in." Repeat on the other side.**

A

B

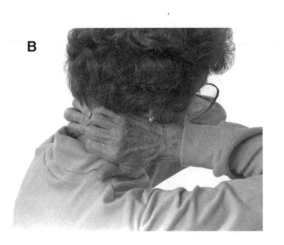

2. **To massage your neck: Rub the right side and back of your neck with your right hand [B]. Use your palm. Rub for at least 30 seconds. Repeat on the left side.**

3. **To massage your lower back:** Place both hands on your lower back and rub firmly up and down all the way to the tailbone, using your whole hand [C].

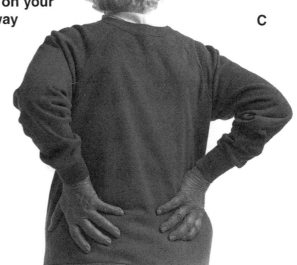

C

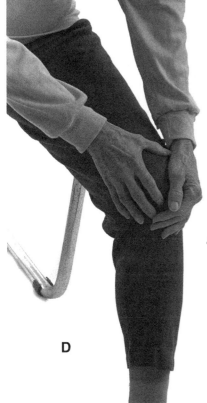

D

4. **To massage your knees:** Massage one knee at a time. Place both hands on your knee. Rub up with one hand and down with the other hand simultaneously in a semicircular motion over the entire knee area [D]. Massage ankles similarly.

5. **To massage your hands:** With your right thumb, rub your left palm and wrist, using a circular motion. Then, starting at the base of your left thumb, use your right thumb on top and right fingers underneath to rub firmly in a circular motion all over and around the joint. Move up the thumb rubbing the same way at each knuckle joint. Repeat with each of your fingers, starting from the base of each [E].

E

FACIAL EXERCISES

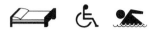

How Will This Exercise Help?

Stretches and tightens facial muscles. Helps lower inhibitions and strengthen vocal cords. Also helps to prevent so-called "monkey lines" around the mouth and nose and make eyes bright, by forcing oxygen into the facial muscles.

Instructors Should Remember...

In the vowel exercise, encourage students to exaggerate the sounds in order to stretch the facial muscles, and to make the vowels as loud as possible.

Verbal Instructions

VOWEL EXERCISE

1. Sit up straight in your chair.

2. Put your hands on your hips.

3. Say AAAAA (as in the word "say") . . . EEEEE . . . IIIII (as in "eye") . . . OOOOO . . . UUUUU ("yooo") [A]. Exaggerate the movement of your lips, jaw, and throat to make the sounds full, round, and rich.

   [Repeat 3 to 5 times.]

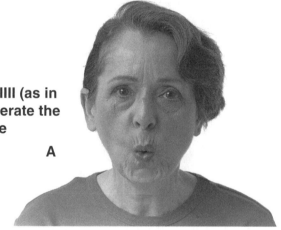

A

CHEEK FILL EXERCISE

1. Sit up straight in your chair. Put your hands on your hips.

2. Look up, fill your cheeks with air, and move the air from side to side and up and down several times, holding your breath in [B].

3. Breathe out and rest for a moment. Then fill your cheeks with air again, hold your breath, and this time move the air around in a circle, two or three times in each direction.

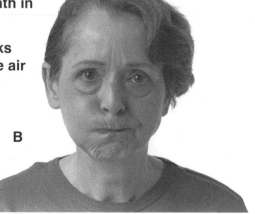

B

EYE EXERCISES

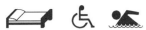

How Will This Exercise Help?

Helps to increase concentration, strengthen the muscles around the eyes, and reduce eyestrain caused by tense muscles. The Eye Palming exercise relieves tension caused by reading, watching television or a computer screen, sewing, or other close work.

Instructors Should Remember . . .

These exercises provide a good focusing routine and are best done just prior to relaxation.

Verbal Instructions

FOCUSING EXERCISE

1. **Hold a pencil or pen (or even your thumb) out at arm's length.**

2. **Focus your eyes on the tip of the pencil [A].**

3. **Now shift your focus to an object at the far end of the room, for example a lamp or picture.**

4. **Shift your focus back and forth from pencil to far wall a few more times. Don't strain.**

5. **Close your eyes and relax.**

Alternative:
Focus your eyes on the pencil and slowly move the pencil in toward your nose, keeping your gaze focused on it the whole time. Then move it slowly back out to arm's length. [Repeat twice more.]

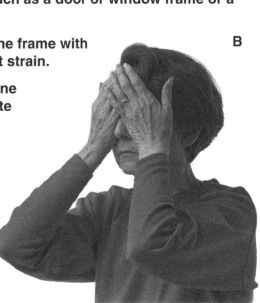

A

B

EYE PATTERNS

1. **Sit comfortably straight in your chair. Choose a space such as a door or window frame or a large object such as a television.**

2. **Starting at one corner of the frame, trace the outline of the frame with your eyes, trying to move your eyes very smoothly. Don't strain.**

3. **Trace a complete pattern around the object or frame in one direction, then reverse and trace the frame in the opposite direction.**

4. **Close your eyes and relax.**

EYE PALMING

1. **To relieve tension around your eyes at any time of day, place your palms gently over your closed eyes and hold for 10 to 30 seconds [B].**

THE LION

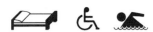

How Will This Exercise Help?	Instructors Should Remember . . .

How Will This Exercise Help?

Invigorates and energizes, while providing emotional release and lowering self-consciousness. Improves the complexion, facial expression, and voice by releasing tension in facial muscles. Helps break the cycle of depression.

Instructors Should Remember . . .

This exercise can "break the ice" because it seems like such a silly exercise; it usually causes some self-conscious laughter which should be encouraged. Participants should be encouraged to "ham it up" and exaggerate movements.

Verbal Instructions

1. Sit up straight with your feet flat on the floor.

2. Spread your fingers apart like a lion's paws and grip your knees.

3. Lean forward slightly and take a deep breath through your nose.

4. Open your eyes wide, raise your eyebrows, stick out your tongue and roar fiercely like a lion!

[Repeat three times.]

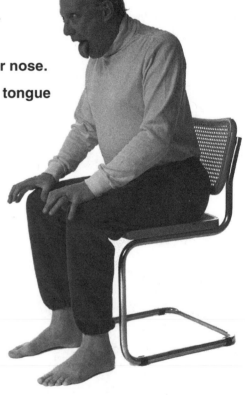

FROG POSE

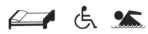

How Will This Exercise Help?

Improves flexibility and circulation in the spine. Improves respiration and also promotes normal bowel function.

Instructors Should Remember . . .

Be sure students move slowly and carefully. The cervical area should especially be bent with care. Everyone can do this exercise, even if they can bend only an inch or two in either direction. Remind students to breathe in and out through the nose.

Verbal Instructions

1. Sit up straight, with your knees slightly separated and your feet flat on the floor. Breathe in and out three times, through your nose.

2. Grasp your knees with your hands.

3. Breathe in deeply as you arch your back and look up, leaning forward slightly [A].

4. Hold your breath [Count to five.]

5. Breathe out as you bend the opposite way, rounding your back and tucking your chin into your chest [B]. Hold your breath. [Count to five.]

6. Relax. How did that feel?

   [Repeat twice more.]

A

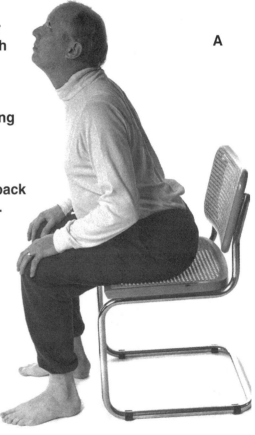

B

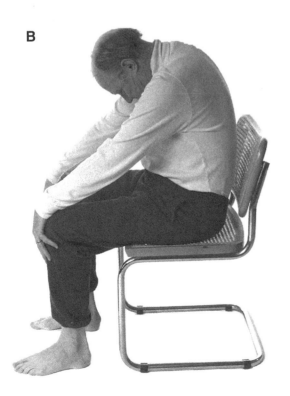

37

SIDE STRETCH

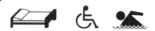

How Will This Exercise Help?

Strengthens muscles and increases lateral mobility of the spine and hip joints. Good for toning of the waistline. Helps breathing problems by stretching and strengthening respiratory muscles.

Instructors Should Remember . . .

Students with weak back and side muscles may have some difficulty at first. Stand close to students to provide support if needed. Remind students to breathe in and out through the nose.

Verbal Instructions

1. **Sit up straight. Let your arms relax at your sides. Breathe in and out three times through your nose.**

2. **Take a deep breath in and bend toward your right side, stretching your right arm down toward the floor and bending your left arm up and over your head.**

3. **Hold your breath.** [Count to three.]

4. **Breathe out and return to the starting position.**

5. **Relax.**

6. **Now switch sides.**

   [Repeat to the left. Rest. Repeat twice more on each side, alternating.]

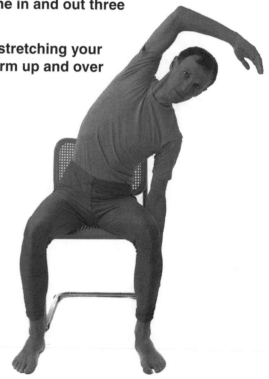

Variations

This exercise can be done in the pool, standing.

SEATED TWIST

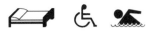

How Will This Exercise Help?

Improves circulation to spine and brain. Improves range of motion in spinal vertebrae. Strengthens shoulder and upper arm muscles. Improves eyesight. The lateral turning motion is important for everyday activities such as looking over one's shoulder when backing up in a car.

Instructors Should Remember . . .

Because this exercise involves a rare lateral movement for most elders, the spinal muscles may feel stiff and/or painful at first. Use extreme caution when teaching this exercise for the first time, and stress small movements in the beginning. Remind students to breathe in and out through the nose.

Verbal Instructions

1. Sit up straight in your chair, with feet flat on the floor. Breathe in and out three times.

2. Place your right hand on the outside of your left knee.

3. Place your left arm across the back of the chair, or inside the back of the chair, or in any comfortable position that pulls the left arm back slightly. Grasp the chair back or seat firmly.

4. Sit up straight, and breathe in completely.

5. Breathe out as you slowly turn toward the left as far as you can. Pull with your right hand to get the greatest stretch. Turn your head as far toward the left as you can, and look to the left with your eyes. Focus on one spot.

6. Hold for a moment. [Count to three.]

7. Now breathe in as you slowly return to face front. Relax.

   [Repeat on the other side. This exercise is done only once in each direction.]

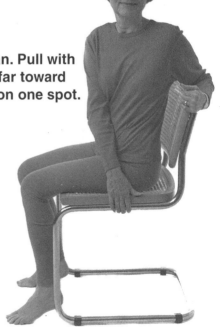

Variations

For students with severe shoulder joint problems, place both hands on the opposite leg instead of twisting one arm behind. This will still strengthen arms and shoulders and provide a gentle twist until the students can manage the complete exercise.

39

SEATED LEG LIFT

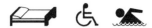

How Will This Exercise Help?

Improves range of motion of the hip joint, strengthens the abdominal, hip, and knee muscles, and stretches the muscles in the back of the legs. Especially useful for improving walking and stair-climbing ability because it strengthens legs and improves balance and confidence.

Instructors Should Remember . . .

Students with arthritis or other problems with the hip joint should start slowly. Avoid painful movements. Emphasize breathing deeply, through the nose, and add repetitions slowly.

Teach the position with hips and back pressed against the chair back to start, as this will provide support for weak back muscles (though the leg will not lift as high in this position; in the completed pose, the thigh should be lifted off the chair seat). After a while, students can try sitting forward slightly, maintaining a straight back during the exercise but not leaning against the chair back. Of course, students with disk or severe muscular problems in the back should use the chair back for support throughout.

 Hip joint and lower back problems.

Verbal Instructions

1. **Sit up straight with hips against the back of your chair, and hold tightly to the side of your chair seat. Breathe in and out three times through your nose.**

2. **Breathe out all your air.**

3. **Now breathe in and hold your breath in as you straighten your right knee and lift your leg to waist level — or as high as you can without straining. Hold.** [Count to three.]

4. **Breathe out as you slowly lower your leg to the floor.**

5. **Relax. How did that feel?**

   [Repeat with the left leg. Rest. Repeat twice more with each leg, alternating.]

6. **Now, sit back in your chair, close your eyes, and try to relax every muscle in your body while you take three slow, gentle breaths.**

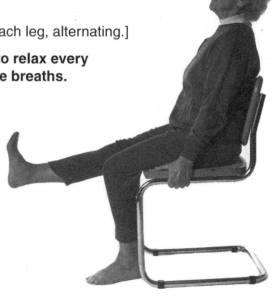

40

Variations

When the above exercise is no longer a challenge for your students, have them try to lift the extended leg up above the level of the chair seat and hold for a count of three.

More frail students should begin with the Foot Flap and Ankle Rotation, as follows. These warm-ups limber and strengthen ankle and calf muscles, and improve circulation in the extremities. They can be done in bed or, for more active students, on the floor.

VARIATION
FOOT FLAP AND ANKLE ROTATION

Verbal Instructions

1. Sit up straight with your hips against the seat back. Hold on to the chair bottom with both hands. Breathe normally throughout this exercise.

2. Stretch your left leg forward and rest the heel on the floor.

3. Gently push your toes forward and pull them back, several times, stretching as far as possible in each direction.

4. Now rotate your ankle, three times in one direction, then three times in the other direction.

5. Rest a moment, then stretch your right foot forward and repeat: toes forward and back several times, then rotate in each direction a few times.

SEATED KNEE SQUEEZE

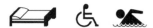

How Will This Exercise Help?

Improves range of motion of the neck, hip, knee, and ankle joints, strengthens the elbow and hip joints, and improves oxygenation of blood. Stretches the muscles and joints used in walking and climbing, as well as muscles in the arms and shoulders used to pull objects. The abdominal smooth muscle tissue is mildly stimulated, and air pressure in the lungs increases slightly during the hold position.

Instructors Should Remember . . .

This exercise is somewhat more strenuous. Be sure you know the medical condition and physical limitations of each participant.

Never exceed three seconds in the holding position, and stress the importance of properly flexing the foot and neck. Do three repetitions with each leg, alternating. Remind students to breathe in and out through your nose.

⊖ Hip, knee, or neck problems; severe hypertension.

Verbal Instructions

1. Sit up straight away from the back of your chair with your arms at your sides. Breathe in and out three times through your nose.

2. Slowly breathe out as much air as possible.

3. Now breathe in, lift your right knee up high, and squeeze it to your chest with both hands.

4. **Hold.** [Count to three.]

5. As you slowly breathe out, relax your arms and lower your leg to the floor.

6. Relax. How did that feel?

   [Repeat with the left leg. Rest. Then repeat twice more with each leg, alternating sides.]

7. Now sit back in your chair, close your eyes, and relax while taking three gentle resting breaths.

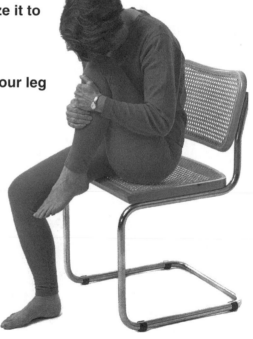

Variations

After your students have mastered the basic technique, have them point their feet and toes down toward the floor. After further practice, during the squeeze, the forehead is lowered toward the knee.

Students with arthritic or painful knee joints may do this exercise grasping underneath their thigh with both hands close to the knee.

LAUGHING BICYCLE

How Will This Exercise Help?

Invigorates and oxygenates the body and brain. Eliminates apathy, depression, and irritability. Increases alertness and interest in life.

Instructors Should Remember . . .

This exercise is usually popular with even the most inhibited students. Be sure to laugh loudly along with your students as you do this exercise with them.

Verbal Instructions

1. Make loose fists and move arms freely in circles as if peddling a bicycle with the hands.

2. Move legs too, leaning back in the chair [A].

3. Laugh out loud for about 30 seconds. Make the sound of laughing and soon you'll really be laughing!

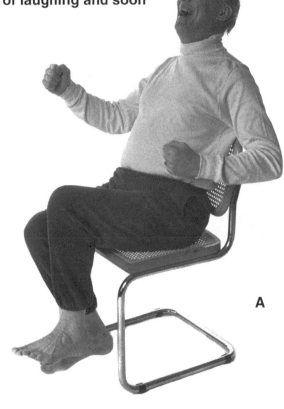

A

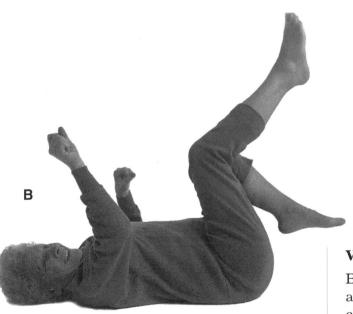

B

Variations

Bedridden clients (or more active clients who are able to get down on the floor easily) can do this exercise lying on their back [B].

FOLDED POSE

How Will This Exercise Help?

Increases range of motion of the neck and back vertebrae; gently stretches the muscles of the neck, back, and hips; and increases blood supply to the head.

This exercise begins to reestablish bending movements important for self-care, and is also important for gradually reducing back pain due to tension or muscular weakness and imbalance, and for pulmonary rehabilitation. With practice, it becomes very relaxing and good for reducing pain in the back and head.

Instructors Should Remember . . .

This movement may cause some anxiety about falling forward in frail students; stand close to students in the beginning. Students with hypertension may experience dizziness or heavy pounding in the temples. Those prone to strokes should be introduced to the exercise very gradually (see variations, below). In the curled position, the pelvis should be slightly extended. All breathing is done through the nose.

⊖ Severe hypertension, spinal problems, stroke.

Verbal Instructions

1. **Sit up straight, with your lower back against the back of your chair.**

2. **Put your knees together, and put your hands on your knees.**

3. **Slowly take in a deep breath through your nose.**

4. **As you slowly breathe out, curl your head and spine toward your knees, bending forward to touch your chest to your thighs.**

5. **If this feels comfortable, let your arms drop to the sides of your legs, hands on the floor. Be sure to let your head and neck relax completely [A].**

6. **Hold.** [Count to three.]

7. **Breathe in and come up slowly, supporting yourself by putting your hands back on your knees. Breathe out.**

8. **Rest and relax. How did that feel?**

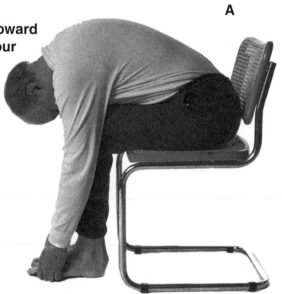

A

Variations

For very frail students, or for those with hypertension who should not lower their head below their heart, substitute the following exercise:

VARIATION

FOLDED POSE VARIATION

Verbal Instructions

1. **Sit up straight, away from the back of your chair. Breathe in and out three times.**

2. **Place hands under your thighs near your knees, and put your knees together.**

3. **Slowly take in a deep breath and hold it.** [Count to three.]

4. **Breathe out as you drop your chin toward your chest and continue curling your spine forward as far as you can** [B]. [This entire movement should take only about 5 seconds.]

5. **Hold your breath out.** [Count to three.]

6. **Now breathe in and straighten, uncurling your spine from the bottom up.**

7. **Relax 30 seconds, breathing normally.**

   [Repeat twice more.]

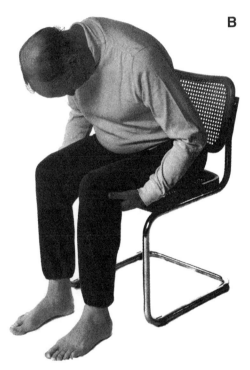

B

SEATED FULL BEND BREATH

How Will This Exercise Help?

Stretches major muscle groups in legs and back, stimulates the breathing and circulatory systems, and improves coordination. Increases overall fitness, helps improve posture, and facilitates bending and reaching movements important for self-care.

Instructors Should Remember . . .

Emphasize a slow breathing pattern to keep pace with the movement of the exercise. Remind students to breathe through their nose always.

Some students may be frightened of losing their balance when bending forward. Make sure legs and feet are firmly in place and that students' hips are against the seat back. In any forward bend, instructors should stand close to the student to give extra support if needed.

Strokes, spine and hip problems, dizziness, pacemakers.

Verbal Instructions

1. **Sit up straight in your chair with knees apart and feet firmly placed on the floor. Rest your lower back against the chair back for support. Breathe in and out three times.**

2. **Breathe out completely, then breathe in as you raise your arms to the sides in a wide circle [A] and overhead [B].**

3. **Look up. Hold.** [Count to three.]

4. **Breathe out as you tuck your head and bend forward slowly, reaching your arms toward the floor. Breathe out all the way forward [C].**

5. **Hold your breath.** [Count to three.]

6. **Slowly breathe in as you raise your arms to the sides and overhead again. Look up.**

7. **Breathe out and relax your arms. Rest. How did that feel?**

   [Repeat twice more.]

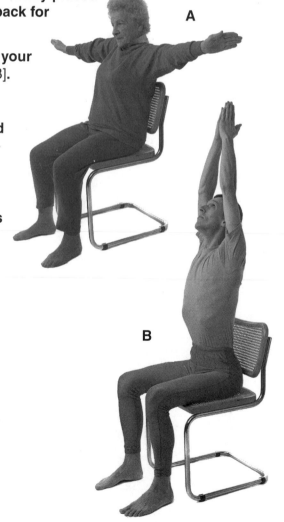

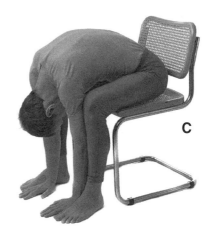

Variations

Frail students can begin with the Supported Full
Bend Breath:

VARIATION
SUPPORTED FULL BEND BREATH

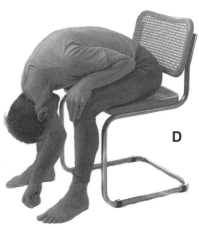

Verbal Instructions

1. Sit straight in your chair with your knees apart and feet firmly
   placed. Breathe in and out three times through your nose.

2. Hold on to your left knee with your left hand. Let your right
   arm hang down at your side.

3. Breathe out completely. Breathe in as you raise your right arm
   up over your head. Make a fist and look up. Hold your breath.
   [Count to three.]

4. As you start to breathe out, tuck your chin and slowly bend
   forward, reaching for the floor with your right hand [D]. Hold your breath out. [Count to three.]

5. Now breathe in and come up, reaching up toward the ceiling with your right arm. Slowly
   breathe out as you lower your arm down to your side.

6. Rest. How did that feel?

   [Repeat on the opposite side. Rest. Repeat twice more on each side, alternating.]

FULL BEND TWIST

How Will This Exercise Help?

Maintains and improves range of motion of the shoulder, torso, and hip joints, strengthens shoulder and upper arm muscles and the oblique muscles of the trunk. Loosens the shoulders and back to facilitate twisting motions, and improves breathing.

Instructors Should Remember . . .

This is an advanced exercise. Emphasize proper breathing and slow, deliberate movements. Know your students' limitations before teaching this exercise. Be sure legs and feet are firmly placed and hips are pressed against the seat back. Stand close to students for support. Remind students to breathe through the nose.

 Spine or shoulder problems.

Verbal Instructions

1. Sit up straight with your arms at your sides and your knees and feet spread apart. Breathe in and out three times through your nose.

2. Breathe out as much as you can.

3. Breathe in deeply as you raise both arms out to the sides and up to shoulder height.

4. Slowly breathe out as you bend forward to touch your RIGHT hand to your LEFT foot [A].

5. Breathe in and come back up straight with arms out to the sides.

6. Breath out and relax your arms. How did that feel?

   [Repeat on the other side. Rest. Repeat twice more on each side, alternating sides.]

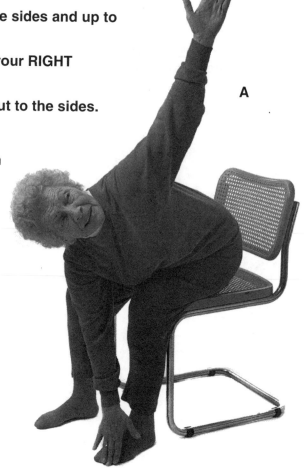

A

Variations

After mastering the above technique, when your students are in the down position, have them look up at the hand that is pointed up toward the ceiling. They should hold the down position for three seconds.

For more frail students, this exercise can be done by holding on with one hand (the Supported Full Bend Twist), instructed as follows:

VARIATION

SUPPORTED FULL BEND TWIST

Verbal Instructions

1. Sit up straight with lower back against the chair back, knees apart and feet firmly placed. Place your left hand on your left knee. Breathe in and out three times.

2. Breathe in as you raise your right arm up and out to the side, shoulder height.

3. Slowly breathe out as you reach down toward your left foot with your right hand [B]. Use your left hand on your knee for support.

4. Slowly breathe in as you come back up.

5. Relax. How did that feel?

   [Repeat on the opposite side. Rest. Repeat twice more on each side, alternating.]

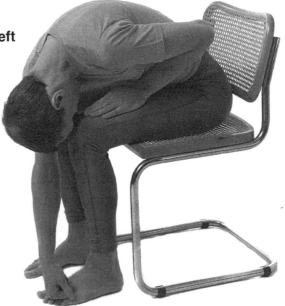

B

ELBOW TO KNEE

How Will This Exercise Help?

Stretches and strengthens back muscles and increases spinal flexibility. Expands chest muscles, which helps to relieve breathing problems.

Instructors Should Remember . . .

Students with weak back muscles or lower back problems need to take extra care with this twisting exercise. Remember to stand close to students to offer support if needed. All breathing should be done through the nose.

⊖ Lower back problems, severe arthritis.

Verbal Instructions

1. **Sit up straight in your chair with your feet flat on the floor about a foot apart. Breathe in and out three times through your nose.**

2. **Clasp your hands behind your neck and breathe in completely** [A].

3. **As you breathe out, bend forward and twist slightly so your right elbow moves toward your left knee** [B].

4. **Hold your breath out.** [Count to three.]

5. **Breathe in and come back up.**

6. **Relax.** [Rest 30 seconds.] **How did that feel?**

   [Repeat on the opposite side. Rest. Repeat twice more on each side, alternating.]

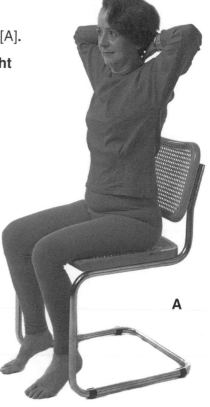

A

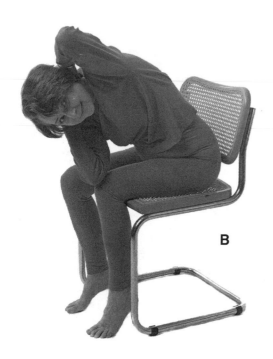

B

Variations

If students cannot reach to clasp their hands behind their neck, they can do this exercise with fingers touching shoulders instead.

SHOULDER TO KNEE

How Will This Exercise Help?

Limbers the spine and strengthens muscles in the back, side, and abdomen. Stimulates and improves functioning of the lungs and kidneys.

Instructors Should Remember . . .

This is a more strenuous version of the Elbow to Knee exercise. The same cautions apply.

Verbal Instructions

1. Sit up straight, away from the back of the chair. Place your feet flat on the floor. Rest your hands on your hips. Breathe in and out three times through your nose.

2. Breathe in completely.

3. Breathe out as you bend forward and lean toward the left, reaching with your right shoulder toward your left knee.

4. Hold your breath. [Count to three.]

5. Breathe in and come up.

6. Relax. How did that feel?

    [Repeat on the opposite side. Rest. Repeat twice more on each side, alternating.]

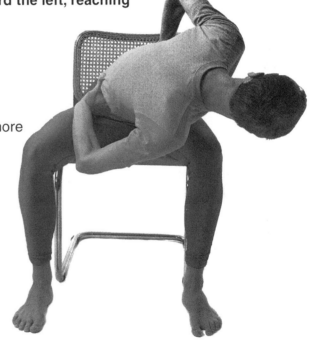

Variations

Students who are afraid of falling may do this exercise holding on to the chair seat at first.

Chapter 4

Standing Exercises

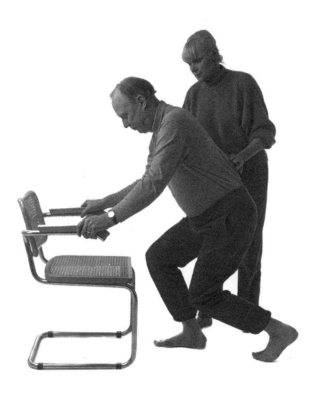

In all standing supported exercises, a barre is ideal, but any sturdy chair on a nonskid surface will do, or even a window sill or counter.

Students will strengthen feet, ankles, and calves more if they practice in bare feet; however, students who feel unbalanced without shoes or who have weak ankles may practice with shoes on at first.

Stand close to and walk among your students to offer support; be especially aware of those frail students who feel unsteady in the balance exercises. Never push students to try a movement they are truly afraid to do; offer an easier variation and let the student gain confidence at his or her own pace. Often, however, if you know your students well, you may know that the student is physically capable of the movement but is reluctant because of, say, an old injury or simply because of habitual inactivity. Gently urge those students to try new movements little by lit-

tle, reinforcing your own confidence in their ability, and soon they will overcome their resistance.

Encourage students to practice the standing exercises at home at any time of day; for instance, while talking on the telephone, students can hold on to a sturdy support and practice the Strut, the Leg Lifts, or a Standing Reach.

Most exercises are done in groups of three repetitions. Always rest 30 seconds after the first repetition of each exercise to be sure students are not straining.

All the standing exercises will strengthen legs and back — essential for getting down on the floor and up again. They build strength and confidence for daily activities such as walking and stair climbing as well.

53

REAR ARM LIFT

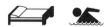

How Will This Exercise Help?

Improves breathing capacity by stretching the muscles of the rib cage, chest, and upper back. Improves posture and helps to straighten rounded shoulders.

Instructors Should Remember . . .

Since this is not a common movement, be careful that students do not strain when doing this exercise for the first time. It will help to do the Shoulder Massage (see page 32) before and after this exercise.

Verbal Instructions

1. **Stand erect, with hands clasped behind your back.**

2. **Breathe out completely through your nose.**

3. **Breathe in as you lift your arms up and away from your body, keeping your hands together.**

4. **Hold.** [Count to three.] **Then breathe out and relax, lowering your arms.**

   [Repeat twice more.]

Variations

Students who are very limber may try to straighten their elbows into a locked position so that the palms are pressed together in back. This is a very difficult movement because it requires great limberness of the shoulders and upper back, but it greatly improves respiration and posture when practiced regularly.

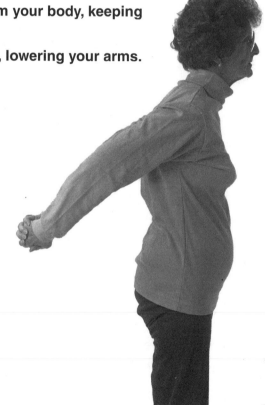

STRUT

do PS '86

How Will This Exercise Help?

Relaxes and invigorates the muscles and joints of the legs, hips, and spine. Strengthens leg muscles for walking, climbing stairs, and is a good preparation for the strength and coordination needed for getting down on the floor and back up safely.

Instructors Should Remember . . .

Encourage students to practice this and the following exercise several times a day to build ankle and leg strength.

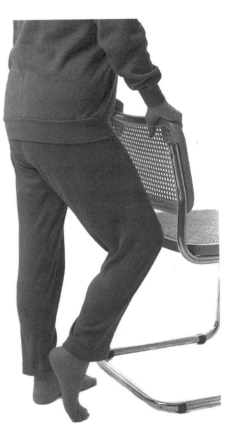

Verbal Instructions

1. Stand behind your chair, holding on with both hands. Your feet should be at a comfortable, stable distance apart. Breathe normally.

2. Keeping the balls and toes of both feet in contact with the floor at all times, bend one knee slightly and then the other, shifting your weight slowly from one side to the other. The spine flexes and the whole body moves gracefully as you strut as if swaying to a slow, dancing beat.

ANKLE STRENGTHENER

How Will This Exercise Help?

Strengthens feet, ankles, and calves, and improves balance; this increases confidence in walking, stair climbing, and other activities.

Instructors Should Remember . . .

Frail students may have difficulty holding the position on their toes at first. Encourage them to hold for a quick three count — even if the time held is only a second.

Verbal Instructions

1. Stand facing a sturdy support such as a barre or chair back, feet together. Hold on with both hands and look straight ahead. Breathe in and out three times through your nose.

2. Breathe in and press up on the toes. Hold the breath and the position. [Count to three.]

3. Breathe out and come back down on flat feet. Rest.

   [Repeat for a total of three to five repetitions.]

do PS. 56

STANDING REACH

How Will This Exercise Help?

Improves balance, posture, and coordination and increases mobility and strength of shoulders and arms. Strengthens ankles and calves, and helps to prevent accidental turning of the ankle while walking. Improves breathing.

Instructors Should Remember . . .

Emphasize no straining or painful lifting of the arms, and have the support at hand in case of loss of balance.

Remind students to stare fixedly at one spot, which will improve balance, and always breathe through the nose.

Verbal Instructions

1. **Stand up straight and breathe gently in and out three times, through your nose.**

2. **Stare at one spot on the wall or floor for balance and breathe out completely.**

3. **Breathe in and raise both your arms to the sides in a wide circle and overhead as high as possible without straining.**

4. **Make fists and push up toward the ceiling. Hold your breath in and look up.** [Count to three.]

5. **Breathe out as you slowly lower your arms to your sides.**

6. **Relax. How did that feel?**

   [Repeat twice more. Remind students to keep staring at one spot for balance.]

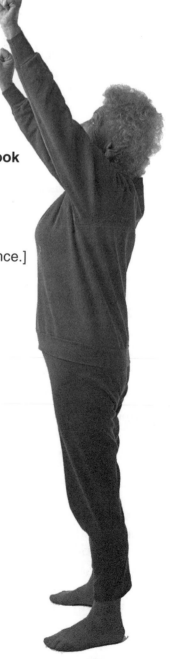

Variations

For more active students: Come up on the toes when breathing in and lifting the arms. Hold to the count of three, then breathe out and come down on the heels while lowering the arms.

Supported Reach: Hold on to the back of the chair or barre with one hand while lifting the other arm and breathing in as above.

Supported Reach on Toes: Hold on to the back of the chair with one hand while lifting the other arm and coming up on the toes. Hold the breath to the count of three and, if possible, look up.

TIP-TOE BALANCE

How Will This Exercise Help?

Maintains and improves range of motion of the ankle, strengthens ankle and calf muscles, and improves balance and coordination. Improves respiration. Strengthens important walking and postural muscles and improves coordination and balance.

Instructors Should Remember . . .

Remind students to stare fixedly at one spot for balance. Fists should be pressed into the soft area of the diaphragm just beneath the rib cage, not on the ribs themselves. Always breathe in and out through the nose.

 Pacemakers, stiff and sore shoulders.

Verbal Instructions

1. **Stand up straight and breathe in and out gently three times through your nose.**

2. **Breathe out completely.**

3. **As you slowly breathe in, rise up on your tip-toes and press your fists into your diaphragm.**

4. **Hold for a moment, staring at one spot on the floor or wall for balance.**
   [Count to three.]

5. **Slowly breathe out as you lower your heels to the floor and arms to your sides.**

6. **Rest and relax. How did that feel?**

   [Repeat twice more.]

Variations

Students who are more frail can hold on to a support with one hand and press in on the diaphragm with one fist only.

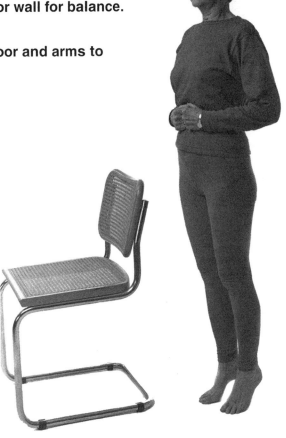

GENTLE FULL BENDS

How Will This Exercise Help?

Increases the range of motion of the shoulders. Provides a whole-body stretch which benefits the nervous and endocrine systems, improves circulation and breathing, and tones muscles.

Instructors Should Remember . . .

Students often try to do this exercise too quickly, like a toe-touch from calisthenics. Emphasize slow, gentle movements done with the breath, always breathing through the nose

 Hypertension, heart disease.

Verbal Instructions

1. **Stand up straight and breathe in and out three times through your nose.**

2. **Breathe in as you lift your arms out to the sides in a wide circle** [A] **and up overhead** [B]. **Look up. Do not strain. Hold.** [Count to three.]

3. **Now slowly breathe out as you bend forward from the waist, tucking your head down** [C].

4. **Hold.** [Count to three.]

5. **Now breathe in deeply as you come back up, arms out to the sides and overhead. Look up at your hands and hold.** [Count to three.]

6. **Breathe out and relax, arms to your sides.**

7. **How did that feel?**

   [Repeat three to five times. Remind students to move slowly, breathing in as they straighten up and breathing out as they bend forward.]

Variations

Frail students can do the Supported Gentle Full Bend exercise holding on to a chair or barre for support (see next page).

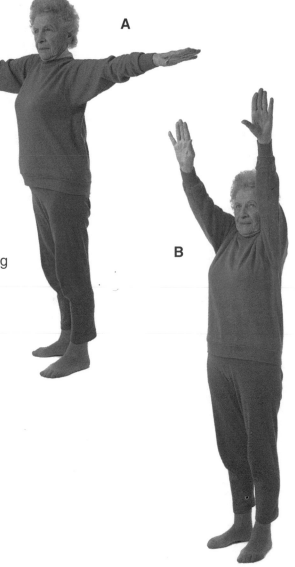

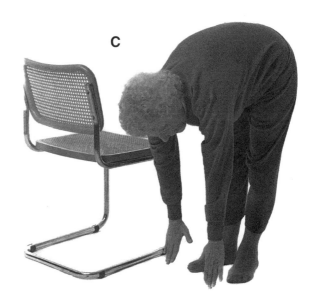

VARIATION
SUPPORTED GENTLE FULL BEND

Verbal Instructions

1. **Hold on to the back of the chair with your left hand.**

2. **Slowly breathe in as you lift your right arm to the side and up, reaching for the ceiling. Look up. Hold.** [Count to three.]

3. **Breathe out as you gently bend from the hips, reaching toward the floor with your right hand. Keep arm and knees straight. It doesn't matter how close to the floor you get. Hold.** [Count to three.]

4. **Breathe in and come back up to a standing position, raising your arm up toward the ceiling again. Hold.** [Count to three.] **Breathe out and lower your arm.**

5. **Rest and relax. How does that feel?**

   [Repeat with other arm.]

STANDING LEG LIFTS

How Will This Exercise Help?

Improves the range of motion of the hip joint and strengthens the muscles of the hips and legs. Helps trim the fatty areas of buttocks and thighs. This exercise is a valuable rehabilitative movement for clients who are recovering from illness or injury and for preventing loss of ambulatory function.

Instructors Should Remember . . .

Be sure to use sturdy supports, especially if you are working with more frail students. A barre attached to the wall is best; a sturdy chair on a non-skid surface will also work. If students seem especially frail or afraid of falling, have them hold on to the chair with both hands instead of one All breathing is done through the nose.

Make sure the torso stays vertical, especially during the extension, and relax for several breaths between each repetition.

 Balance problems, weak ankles, hip problems.

○ Verbal Instructions

1. **Stand up straight and to the right of your support and hold tightly with your left hand. Place your right hand on your hip. Breathe in and out slowly three times through your nose.**

2. **Now, breathe out completely.**

3. **Breathe in and lift your right leg straight up in front. Hold the position and your breath.** [Count to three.]

4. **Breathe out and lower the leg back to the floor. Rest and relax. Shake out your leg.**

5. **Breathe in and lift your right leg straight out to the side. Hold the position and your breath.** [Count to three.]

6. **Breathe out and lower it back to the floor. Rest and relax. Shake out your leg.**

7. **Breathe in and lift your right leg straight out in back. Hold the position and your breath.** [Count to three.]

8. **Breathe out and lower it back down to the floor. Shake out your leg.**

9. **Rest and relax. How did that feel?**

   [Repeat with the left leg, holding on with the right hand.]

10. **Now, relax all the muscles in your back, hips, belly, and legs as**

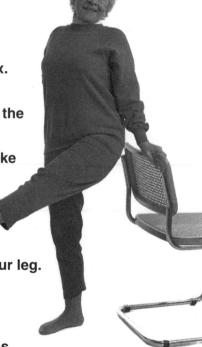

Variations

Students with very weak leg and back muscles should begin by holding for a shorter count and slowly working to increase the time held.

STANDING KNEE SQUEEZE

How Will This Exercise Help?

Helps develop balance and concentration. Strengthens the arms and shoulders, legs, and feet, and improves circulation and digestion.

Instructors Should Remember . . .

Do not attempt the more advanced variation until students are quite strong in the supported version. Those with arthritis or other joint problems in their knees can grasp underneath the thigh near the knee. All breathing is done through the nose.

Verbal Instructions

1. **Stand straight, holding on to a chair or barre for support with your right hand. Breathe gently in and out three times through your nose.**

2. **Breathe in deeply as you raise your left knee in front of you.**

3. **Wrap your left arm around your knee and hold your breath and the position as you gently squeeze the knee toward your chest.**

4. **Bend your head toward your knee slightly.** [Count to three.]

5. **Breathe out as you relax and lower your leg to the floor.**

6. **Relax. How did that feel?**

   [Repeat on the opposite side. Rest. Repeat twice more on each side, alternating, for a total of three times on each leg.]

Variations

When students attain greater strength and balance they can do this exercise with both arms wrapped around the knee. Remind them to stare at one spot for balance.

SIMPLE ALTERNATE TRIANGLE

How Will This Exercise Help?

Stretches back of legs and lower back. Improves mobility of hips, shoulders, and spine. Stimulates circulation throughout the body and brain. May help relieve depression.

Instructors Should Remember . . .

Rest after each two repetitions (one to each side). Check for mid-back pain, and for stiffness the day after doing the exercise. Breathe through the nose at all times.

 Lower back or hip problems.

Verbal Instructions

1. Stand with your feet apart a comfortable distance apart and toes pointed toward the front.

2. Breathe in completely as you lift your arms and open them wide to the sides to shoulder height.

3. Breathe out as you slowly bend toward one leg and grasp your leg with both hands as far down the leg as you can comfortably. Pull gently by bending your elbows. Hold your breath out. [Count to three.]

4. Now breathe in and come up, opening your arms out to shoulder height.

5 Breathe out and lower your arms.

6. Relax. How did that feel?

   [Repeat on the other side. Rest. Repeat twice more to each leg for a total of three repetitions to each leg.]

Variations

Students who are unsure of their balance may do this exercise holding on with one hand to a barre or chair back for support.

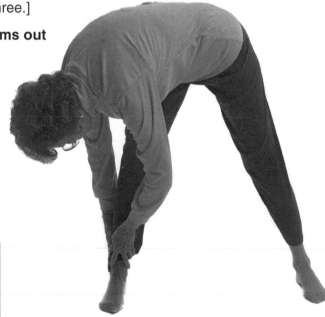

TREE POSE

How Will This Exercise Help?

Develops concentration, poise, and balance. Strengthens leg muscles and promotes a healthy, strong nervous system.

Instructors Should Remember . . .

An important technique in this exercise is the ability to relax the stomach and breathing muscles. Since most people tend to hold their breath while trying to balance on one leg, even while supported, you should constantly remind your students to relax their breath. Another common mistake students make is to try to leap to the full balance position all at once. It is much better to balance at each step first. Remind students to stare at one spot, which will also help balance.

Many people have trouble finding a comfortable place to rest their lifted foot on the opposite leg. Most people have success if they "hook" the foot over the opposite knee joint. Remind students to let their lifted leg relax and it will stay in place better. It also helps to do this exercise in bare feet.

Verbal Instructions

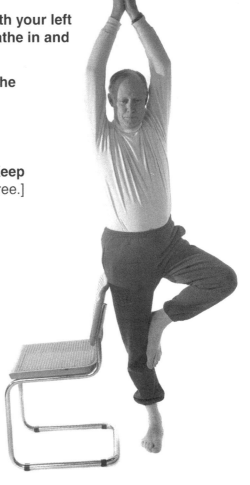

1. **Stand straight, holding on to the back of a chair or barre with your left hand for support. Stare at one spot for balance. Gently breathe in and out three times through your nose.**

2. **Breathe normally as you lift your right foot and place it on the inside of your left leg, as high up as you can. Let your right (lifted) leg relax and it will stay in place better.**

3. **Keep staring at one spot and breathing normally.**

4. **When you feel steady, slowly lift your right arm overhead. Keep staring at one spot and relax your breath. Hold.** [Count to three.]

5. **Relax and lower your arm and leg.**

   [Repeat on the opposite side.]

Variations

When students are confident with this exercise, they can try lifting both arms overhead in Step 5, as in the illustration.

REAR LEG LIFTS and SUPER BALANCE POSE

How Will This Exercise Help?

Strengthens legs, hips, and back muscles, limbers hip joints, improves balance and concentration, and improves circulation to the extremities. Increases confidence.

Instructors Should Remember . . .

Encourage students to lift the back leg parallel to the floor without straining. Many students have a tendency to bend either or both legs as they lift. Encourage them to keep the knees straight, but not locked. All breathing is done through the nose.

Verbal Instructions

REAR LEG LIFTS

1. **Stand facing the back of your chair and hold on with both hands. Be sure you have enough room in back of you to raise your leg without hitting another student.**

2. **Step back from the chair so you are leaning forward slightly.**

3. **Breathe out completely. Now breathe in and slowly lift your right leg in back as high as you can without strain** [A]. **Keep both legs straight. Hold.** [Count to three.]

4. **Breathe out and lower the leg. How did that feel?**

   [Repeat on left leg. Rest. Repeat twice more on each side, alternating legs.]

5. **Rest a moment, then try the Super Balance Pose.**

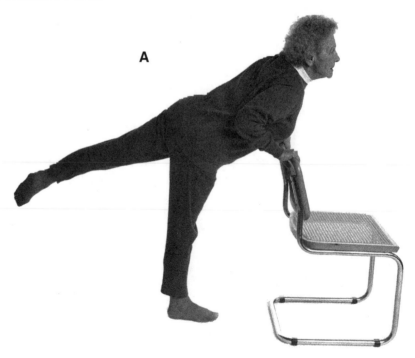

A

Verbal Instructions

SUPER BALANCE POSE

1. Hold on to the chair with both hands and step back a little so you are leaning forward.

2. Breathe normally — don't hold your breath.

3. Slowly lift your right leg in back, keeping both legs straight.

4. Hold the position, breathing normally, and slowly loosen your grip on the chair. Do not let go completely! If you feel really steady, you can straighten your arms just above the chair [B], but be ready to hold on again immediately if you feel unsteady. Look forward across your outstretched hands. Remember to keep breathing normally.

5. Now grasp the chair again, lower your leg, and relax. How did that feel?

   [Rest a few moments and repeat on the other side. This exercise should be done only once on each side.]

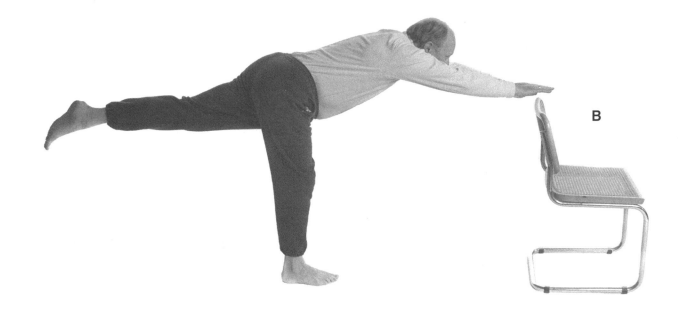

B

CHAPTER 5

FLOOR EXERCISES

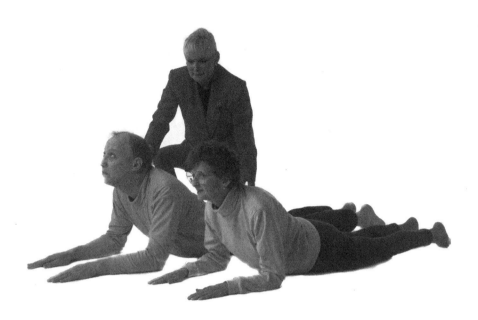

The ability to get down on the floor and back up easily is one of the most important techniques that Easy Does It Yoga offers. Someone who cannot do this will always be limited in their physical activity. They will always be afraid of falling and not being able to get up; they will be fearful of being alone for the same reason; and they will feel frustrated at not being able to perform simple daily tasks such as cleaning a bottom shelf or picking up their glasses that have dropped to the floor.

In over 20 years of teaching this program, we have found only a few students who were unable to learn this technique: those with chronic, painful knee joint problems affecting both knees, and those whose arms were too weak. Most students are not only able but very excited about learning a technique that frees them from fear and dependence.

There are several preparatory exercises that strengthen the arms and legs and practice the coordination of the various movements needed in this technique. With frail students, you may need to practice these exercises for several weeks before attempting to get down on the floor.

You will have most success if you work with each student individually on this technique. It is important to pay attention to details such as the distance the student stands from the chair as he or she begins. You should be right there to make sure their first experience is a successful one, and they need to know that your hand is there to support them if they do not feel secure at first.

Once students have mastered the technique, they can begin to practice some of the Easy Does It exercises in this section that are done on the floor. (Remember that most of these can also be done in bed; a special symbol indicates these.) Start with the seated positions and slowly work into the lying down positions. To move from a seated to a lying down position, tell students to rest on one elbow, supporting their weight with their opposite hand, and then to slowly lower themselves onto their back. To get back up to a seated position, roll to one side, place one hand in back for support, roll up on one elbow, then push up to a seated position.

Floor exercises will be more comfortable if students practice on a soft mat or blanket. A thin foam mat is also suitable.

LAZY KNEE BENDS

How Will This Exercise Help?

Strengthens knees and ankles in preparation for getting down on the floor without strain.

Instructors Should Remember . . .

Be sure students keep the torso straight while bending the knees; otherwise their back works instead of their legs.

Verbal Instructions

1. There are two parts to this exercise. First, to warm up, just hold on to the chair with both hands and slowly bend your knees — just a few inches at first. Keep your feet flat on the floor. Breathe normally throughout this exercise.

   [Repeat several times.]

2. Now stand away from the chair and place your hands firmly on your knees.

3. Gently bend and straighten your knees as before, keeping your feet flat. Don't bend too far. Keep your hands on your knees for support.

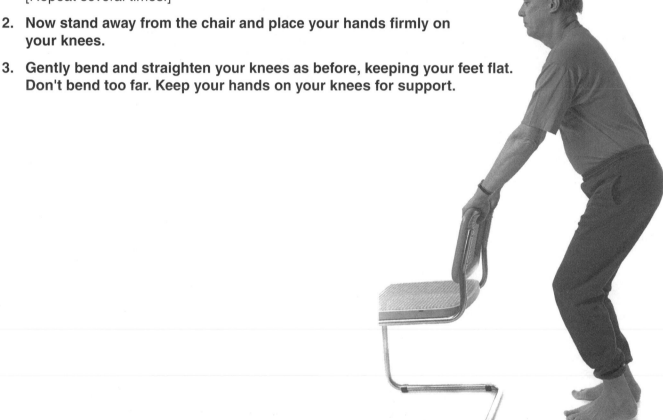

LEG AND ARM STRENGTHENERS

How Will This Exercise Help?

Builds upper arm and shoulder strength to help in the technique of getting down to the floor and back up safely.

Instructors Should Remember . . .

Encourage students to practice both variations of this exercise at home several times a day for quicker results.

Many students have a tendency to place their feet away from the chair, making it harder to bend the knees and causing more strain on the arms. One foot should always be close to the front chair leg; when the front knee bends, the knee should extend slightly out to one side, not straight forward into the chair. Work with each student individually for best results.

As you repeat this exercise, gradually have students bend further down until they can rest one knee on the floor and push themselves back into a standing position. They will then be ready to move on to the actual technique of getting down to the floor.

Verbal Instructions

1. **Stand facing your chair. Lean forward and grasp the sides of the chair seat firmly with both hands.**

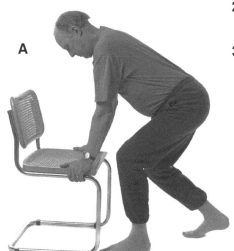

A

2. **Place your left foot near the left front leg of the chair, and your right foot behind you.**

3. **Leaning on your hands, slowly bend your knees, keeping your weight on your hands, and then use your hands to push yourself back up. Bend as far as you can and still straighten up again** [A].

[Repeat with the right foot forward near the right front leg of the chair.]

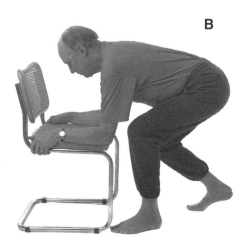

B

Variations

When students become stronger, do the same exercise with the forearms resting on the seat of the chair and elbows bent [B].

69

GETTING DOWN ON THE FLOOR

How Will This Exercise Help?

Getting down on the floor and back up safely improves self-esteem by allowing students to do many household chores by themselves. It relieves anxiety about what would happen if they fell and could not get help right away. It also builds physical strength and stamina which creates feelings of well-being and a sense of independence.

Instructors Should Remember . . .

This technique normally is learned over a period of several weeks, depending on how often the class meets, how motivated students are to practice at home between class meetings, and how frail students are to begin with. You should allow enough time to work individually with as many students as possible. To ensure that chairs won't slip, push them against the wall. Stop frequently to ask how students are feeling. Be sure to try the technique yourself before you teach it.

Students who have one knee with arthritis or other joint problems that would make putting weight on the joint painful should make sure that they bend with the other (good) knee toward the floor. A pad of foam rubber in front of the chair on the floor will also help to protect the knees.

Some students may have better luck supporting themselves with their forearms instead of just their hands in the reverse (getting up) sequence.

Verbal Instructions

1. **Stand facing the front of a sturdy chair, bend at the waist, and grasp the outside edges of the chair seat firmly** [A].

2. **Place your right foot near the right front chair leg and your left foot slightly behind you.**

3. **Using your arms for support, bend your knees and slowly lower your left knee toward the floor** [B].

A

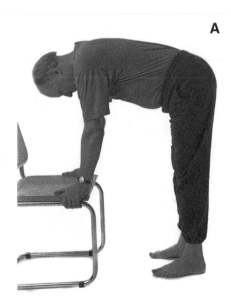

B

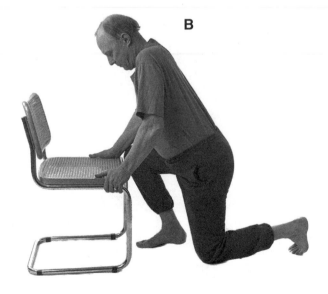

4. Continuing to hold on to the chair seat for support, slowly lower your right knee to the floor [C].

5. Hold on to the chair with your right hand and carefully place your left hand on the floor near your left hip [D].

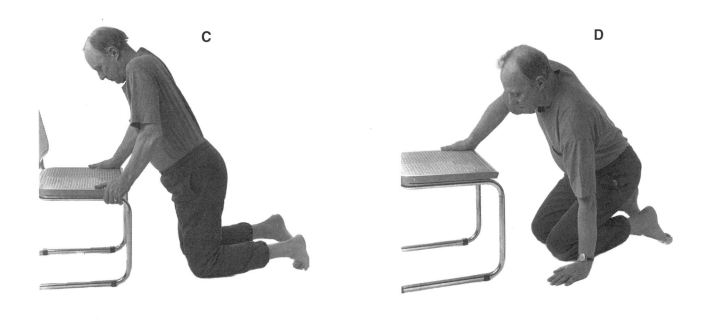

6. Shifting your weight to your left arm, carefully bring your right hand down to the floor on your left side. Lean on both hands [E].

7. Supporting your weight on both hands, slowly lower your hips toward the floor near your left hand [F].

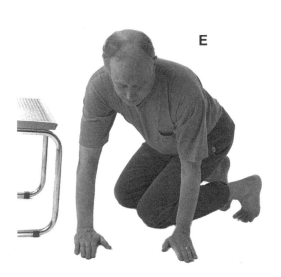
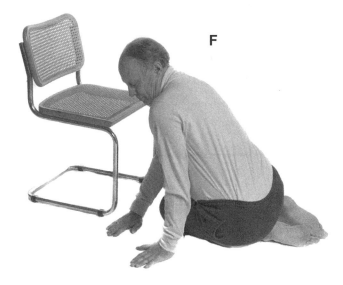

8. Bring your hands around to support you in back and slowly straighten your right leg [G].

9. Now unfold your left leg so you are sitting with both legs outstretched, leaning on your hands [H].

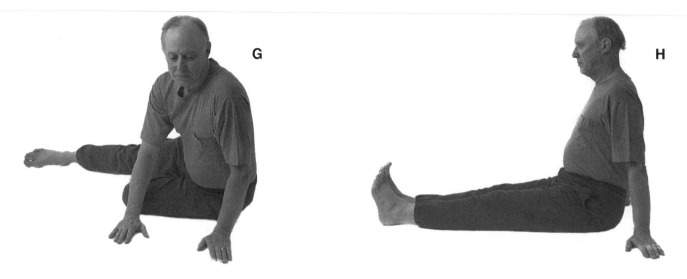

Verbal Instructions

TO GET UP FROM THE FLOOR

1. Starting from a seated position with legs outstretched, bend both knees and let your legs bend toward the right.

2. Place both hands next to your right hip.

3. Carefully push yourself up on your hands and knees, using your arms.

4. Walk on all fours over to a sturdy chair.

5. Lift your left hand and grasp the side of the chair seat firmly.

6. Grasp the right side of the chair seat with your right hand, and move forward on your knees so you are close to the chair. Tuck your toes under.

7. Carefully raise your left foot and place it flat on the floor.

8. Putting your weight on your arms, push yourself up so you are standing on both feet.

9. Slowly stand up.

SUN POSE STRETCH

How Will This Exercise Help?

Prepares the student to do the Seated Sun Pose, by gently introducing the movements in a non-strenuous warm-up while stretching and strengthening the lower back. Helps prevent sciatica, improves digestion, and stimulates circulation in vital organs.

Instructors Should Remember . . .

Students with lower back problems should be very careful not to stretch forward too far in this exercise because of the danger of pulling the lower back muscles. Remind students to breathe in and out through the nose.

Verbal Instructions

1. **Sit straight with legs outstretched. Place your hands under your legs near your knees.**

2. **Take a deep breath in as you arch your back, look up, and pull your upper body slightly toward your legs by bending your elbows** [A].

3. **Breathe out as you round your back and tuck your head forward** [B]. **Hold your breath out.** [Count to three.]

4. **Breathe in and sit up. Relax. How did that feel?**

   [Repeat twice more.]

Variations

This exercise can be done sitting up in bed with the lower back supported by the headboard.

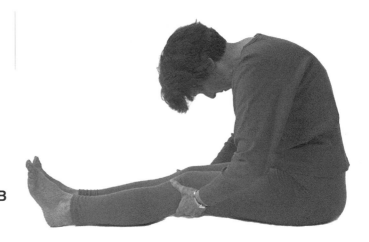

A

B

73

SEATED SUN POSE

How Will This Exercise Help?

Strengthens abdominal muscles, improves digestion and breathing, stretches and strengthens legs and spine. May help prevent sciatica.

Instructors Should Remember . . .

To help prevent cramps, rest frequently and always do Foot Flaps and Ankle Rotations (see p. 41) before this exercise. All breathing is done through the nose.

Note that this exercise uses two complete breath cycles. Be sure students complete the pose (arms to sides: Step 5 below) and rest for at least 30 seconds before repeating the exercise.

 Lower back problems.

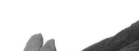

1. Sit straight with legs outstretched. Breathe in and out three times through your nose.

2. Breathe out completely. Breathe in as you raise your arms in a wide circle and over your head. Look up and hold [A]. [Count to three.]

3. Breathe out as you tuck your head and bend forward over your legs. Grasp your legs underneath firmly and bend your elbows, pulling your upper body toward your legs [B]. **Hold.** [Count to three.]

4. Release and start to breathe in as you raise your arms in another wide circle overhead. Look up.

5. Breathe out and relax, arms to sides. Rest. [Pause 30 seconds.] **How did that feel?**

A

Variations

This exercise can be done sitting up in bed with the lower back supported by the headboard.

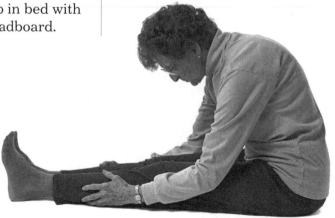

B

EASY ALTERNATE SUN POSE

How Will This Exercise Help?

Same benefits as the Seated Sun Pose. Additionally, this exercise stretches the groin muscles and limbers the knee joints.

Instructors Should Remember . . .

Students with arthritic or painful knees should bend the leg only as far as is comfortable and place a pillow under the bent knee. All students should massage the knees before and after the exercise (see p. 33). All breathing is done through the nose.

 Severe arthritic knees, lower back problems.

Verbal Instructions

1. **Sit straight with legs together. Bend your left leg and place your left foot flat as high up on the inside of your right leg as you can without straining. Breathe in and out three times through your nose.**

2. **Breathe out completely, then breathe in as you raise your arms in a wide circle to the sides and overhead. Look up [A]. Hold.** [Count to three.]

3. **Breathe out as you tuck your head and bend forward over your right leg. Grasp your leg underneath firmly and bend your elbows, pulling your upper body toward your leg [B]. Hold.** [Count to three.]

4. **Release and start to breathe in as you raise your arms in another wide circle overhead. Look up. Hold.** [Count to three.]

5. **Breathe out and relax, arms to sides. Rest.** [Pause 30 seconds.] **How did that feel?**

[Repeat twice more for a total of three repetitions. Straighten the leg and massage the knee. Repeat three times on opposite side.]

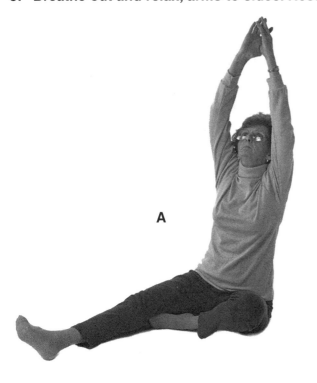

A

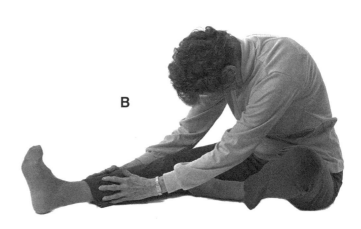

B

GENTLE TWIST

How Will This Exercise Help?

Improves flexibility of the spine and increases circulation to the brain. Helps in daily activities such as being able to turn around while backing up a car. Also strengthens shoulder and arm muscles, and improves memory, eyesight, and breathing.

Instructors Should Remember . . .

It is most important for the spine to remain straight while turning in order to get a true sideways twist. The hand in back should be as close to the body as possible, fingers pointed in. The student should look around behind as far as possible. All breathing is done through the nose.

 Spinal disk problems.

Verbal Instructions

1. Sit straight with legs together, pointed front. Toes should be pointed toward the ceiling. Breathe in and out three times through your nose.

2. Place your right hand across your left thigh and place your left hand in back of you, palm down, fingers pointing in toward your back. Place the palm as close to your body as you can.

3. Sit up straight and look forward. Breathe in completely.

4. Breathe out as you slowly turn and look back over your left shoulder. Use your arms to pull and push yourself around as far as you can without straining.

5. Look at a spot on the wall at eye level with your eyes as far left as you can see.

6. Hold this position, breathing gently, for a moment or two. [Count to three or five.]

7. Breathe in, release, and turn back to the front. Relax.

8. How did that feel?

9. Now repeat on the other side: Place your left hand across your right thigh and your right hand in back on the floor.

10. Breathe in completely, then breathe out as you turn toward the right, looking over your right shoulder and gazing at a spot on the wall at eye level as far toward the right as possible without straining.

11. Hold, breathing gently. [Count to three or five.]

12. Return to face front and relax.

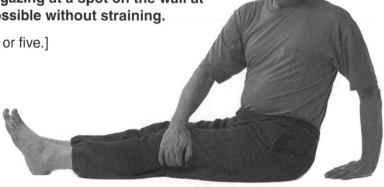

ALTERNATE TORTOISE STRETCH

How Will This Exercise Help?

Improves circulation to pelvic region, stretches nerves and muscles in legs and ankles, limbers lower back, and helps prevent prostate problems.

Instructors Should Remember . . .

Students with lower back or sciatica problems should be very careful when bending forward. Have all students begin by reaching down only as far as their knees at first. Remind students to always breathe through the nose.

 Lower back problems.

Verbal Instructions

1. **Sit straight and separate your legs as far as you can. Your toes should be pointed toward the ceiling. Breathe in and out three times.**

2. **Breathe out completely, then breathe in deeply as you raise your arms in a circle to the sides and overhead. Look up. Hold.** [Count to three.]

3. **Breathe out as you bend toward your right leg, tucking your head. Grasp your right leg firmly and bend your elbows to pull your upper body toward your leg. Do not strain! Hold.** [Count to three.]

4. **Release your leg, breathe in deeply, and come back up, bringing your arms in another wide circle to the sides and overhead. Look up. Hold.** [Count to three.]

5. **Breathe out and lower your arms. Rest.** [Pause 30 seconds.] **How did that feel?**

   [Repeat to the left side. Rest. Repeat twice more to each leg, alternating sides.]

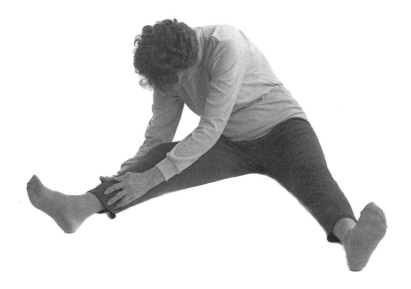

KNEE SQUEEZE

How Will This Exercise Help?

Limbers the back and hips, relieves lower back tension, strengthens abdominal muscles, and improves digestive function and breathing.

Instructors Should Remember . . .

Students with lower back problems should begin with knees bent and feet on the floor a few inches apart.

Note that in this exercise, unlike most others in the program, the breath comes IN as the body is compressed; this is essential for the effectiveness of the exercise. The breath should be held in to a count of three, and then expelled slowly in a controlled manner. Remember that all breathing is done through the nose.

Verbal Instructions

1. **Lie on your back with arms at your sides and legs together. Breathe in and out three times.**

2. **Breathe out completely.**

3. **Breathe in as you bend your right knee and grasp it with both hands, bringing it in toward your chest.**

4. **Hold your breath in as you squeeze your knee to your chest and lift your forehead up toward your knee** [A]. [Count to three.]

5. **Relax and breathe out as you lower your head, arms, and legs down to the floor. How did that feel?**

6. **Repeat with the left leg: Breathe out completely. Breathe in as you bend your left knee and grasp it with both hands, bringing it in toward your chest. Hold your breath in as you squeeze your knee to your chest and lift your forehead up toward your knee. Relax and breathe out.**

   [Repeat twice more on each side, alternating.]

A

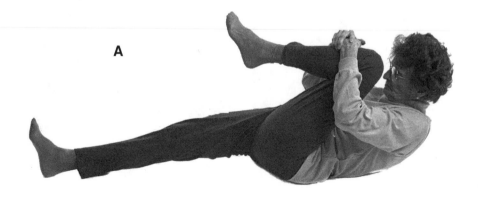

Variations

Double Knee Squeeze: Start with both legs bent unless students are quite strong. Exercise sequence is the same, but students should wrap their arms around both knees to squeeze [B], and should return legs to the bent-knee position unless they are strong enough to straighten the legs without straining their lower back.

In both variations of this exercise, students with arthritic or painful knees may grasp the legs underneath their thighs close to the knees.

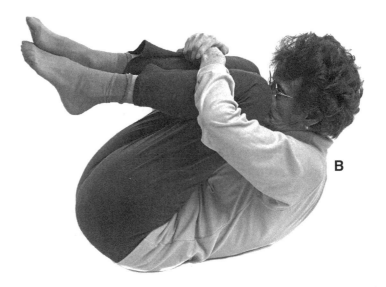

B

EASY BRIDGE

How Will This Exercise Help?

Improves functioning of thyroid and entire endocrine system, relieves lower back pain and fatigue, improves complexion by bringing circulation to the head, and helps relieve bedsores.

Instructors Should Remember . . .

This exercise should be done as a half lift, not a full arched bridge, which puts much more stress on the back of the neck. All breathing is done through the nose.

 Cervical spine problems.

Verbal Instructions

1. Lie on your back and bend your knees. Place your feet several inches apart as close to your hips as possible. Lay your arms palms down at your sides. Breathe in and out three times through your nose.

2. Breathe out completely. Relax your shoulders.

3. Breathe in slowly as you raise your hips off the floor, curling your spine up to your waist. Your waist should remain on the floor.

4. Hold the position and your breath for a moment.

5. Breathe out as you slowly lower your hips to the floor.

6. Relax. How did that feel?

[Repeat twice more.]

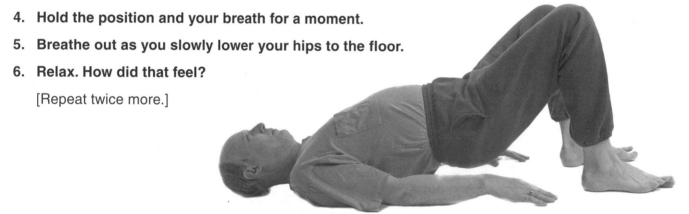

Variations

When students get much stronger, and if they have no cervical problems, they may try a full arched pose: The hips are raised higher and the back arched as much as possible so that the chin is tucked into the chest.

ALTERNATE TOE TOUCH

How Will This Exercise Help?

Stretches and strengthens the muscles and joints of the legs, hips, and lower back; helps relieve sciatica.

Instructors Should Remember . . .

Both knees should remain straight, even if it means the student cannot touch the toe at first. Always breathe in and out through the nose.

Verbal Instructions

1. **Lie on your back with your legs straight, right arm over your head, and left arm at your side. Breathe in and out three times through your nose.**

2. **Breathe out completely, then breathe in as you lift your right arm and right leg simultaneously.**

3. **Reach toward your toe, but keep your shoulders on the floor.**

4. **Don't bend your knees — it's more important to keep your knees straight than to touch your toe. Hold.** [Count to three.]

5. **Breathe out and relax, bringing your right arm down to the floor over your head. How did that feel?**

6. **Now bring your right arm down and lift the left arm over your head to do the exercise on the opposite side.**

   [Repeat twice more on each side, alternating.]

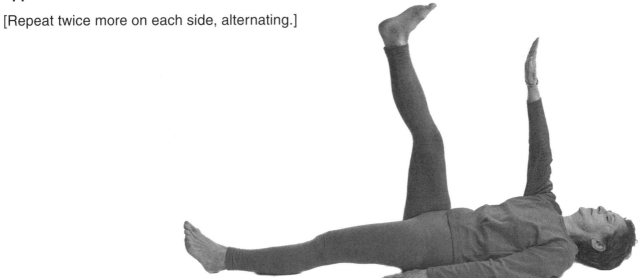

Variations

Students who have very weak hip and leg muscles may begin the exercise with legs bent and feet flat on the floor.

LOWER BACK STRETCH

How Will This Exercise Help?

Improves functioning of internal organs. Improves circulation. Strengthens and limbers the shoulders, back, and hip joints. Helps to trim the waistline.

Instructors Should Remember . . .

Students with disk problems in their lower back should be very careful with this exercise. All breathing is done through the nose.

 Spinal disk problems.

Verbal Instructions

1. Lie on your back with your legs together and arms stretched out to the sides, palms down. Breathe in and out three times through your nose.

2. Breathe out, then breathe in as you lift your left leg and hook your left toe under your right knee.

3. Breathe out as you bend your left leg to the right over your right leg toward the floor as far as possible without straining. Keep your shoulders and arms on the floor and keep your right leg straight.

4. Hold the position and your breath. [Count to three.]

5. Breathe in as you roll back, lift your left knee up, and straighten your leg toward the ceiling.

6. Breathe out as you return the leg to the floor.

7. How did that feel?

   [Rest 30 seconds. Repeat with right leg. Rest and relax. Repeat twice more on each side, alternating.]

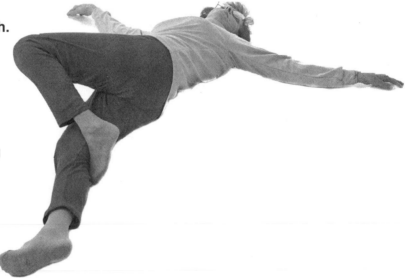

EASY COBRA LIFT

How Will This Exercise Help?

Limbers and strengthens spinal column and back muscles. Strengthens upper back and shoulders. Improves breathing.

Instructors Should Remember . . .

Be sure students are in the correct position to start this exercise: elbows close in to the body, shoulders relaxed, head relaxed. All breathing is done through the nose.

 Spinal disk problems.

Verbal Instructions

1. **Lie on your stomach and raise your body on your elbows, with the elbows close in to the body. Position your arms so that your elbows and shoulders are in a straight line up and down. Place your hands palms down in front of you. Let your forehead relax toward the floor and relax your shoulders** [A].

2. **Breathe out completely, then breathe in as you slowly lift your head and stretch up and back without lifting your elbows off the floor. Look up through your forehead** [B]. **Hold.**
   [Count to three.]

3. **Breathe out and slowly drop your forehead toward the floor and relax. Rest. How did that feel?**

   [Repeat twice more.]

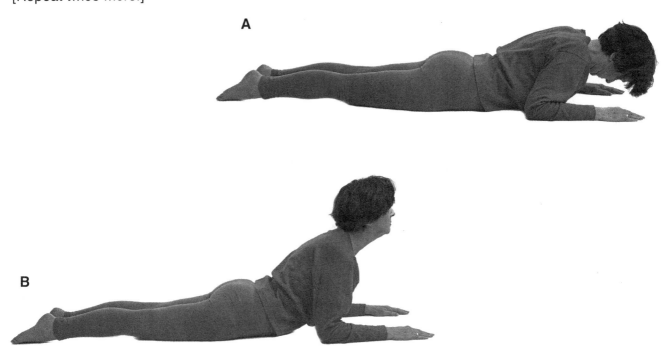

A

B

BACK STRENGTHENERS

How Will This Exercise Help?

Strengthens both sides of the back evenly. Stimulates circulation throughout the extremities and strengthens arms, shoulders, hips, and thighs.

Instructors Should Remember . . .

Keeping the legs straight while lifting is more important than lifting high. Some students may be able to lift only an inch or two at first; even this will gradually build strength. Encourage students to practice this exercise every day. Remind students to always breathe through the nose.

Verbal Instructions

1. **Lie on your stomach with your forehead on the floor and arms at your sides. Make fists. Breathe in and out three times through your nose.**

2. **Breathe out completely. Breathe in as you lift your right leg in back, keeping it straight** [A]. **Hold.** [Count to three.]

3. **Breathe out and lower the leg. Rest and relax. How did that feel?** [Rest 30 seconds.]

   [Repeat with left leg. Rest. Repeat twice more on each side, alternating.]

4. **After a rest, come back into position with your forehead on the floor and stretch your arms in front of you on the floor.**

5. **Breathe out completely, then breathe in as you lift arms, head, and legs, keeping them straight** [B]. **Look up. Hold.** [Count to three.]

6. **Breathe out and lower to the floor. Relax. Rest.** [Pause 30 seconds.]

   [Repeat twice more, resting between each repetition.

A

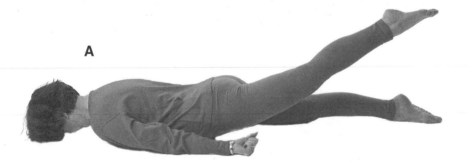

B

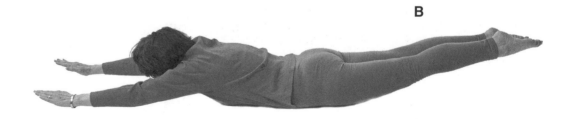

ALL FOURS LIFT

How Will This Exercise Help?

Strengthens shoulders, back, and hip joints; improves balance and posture.

Instructors Should Remember . . .

To help with balance, have students stare at one spot on the floor in front. In Part 2 of this exercise (steps 5–7), many students tend at first to try to lift the arm and leg on the same side of the body (which is a more difficult variation) instead of opposites. All breathing is done through the nose.

 Lower back problems, arthritic knees.

Verbal Instructions

1. **Come up to your hands and knees and look straight ahead. Breathe in and out three times through your nose.**

2. **Breathe out completely, then breathe in as you straighten your right leg and lift it up in back as high as you can** [A]. **Look up slightly and hold.** [Count to three.]

3. **Lower your leg as you breathe out.**

4. **Rest. How did that feel?**

   [Repeat with left leg. Rest. Repeat twice more on each leg, alternating.]

5. **Come back to your starting position. Breathe out.**

6. **As you breathe in, slowly lift your RIGHT arm and your LEFT leg (opposites)** [B]. **Stare at one spot on the wall for balance. Hold.** [Count to three.]

7. **Breathe out and lower your arm and leg. Rest. How did that feel?**

   [Repeat with left arm and right leg. Rest. Repeat twice more on each side, alternating.]

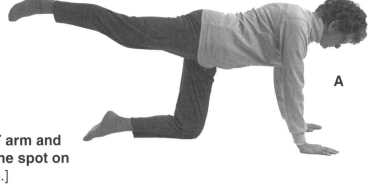

A

Variations

When balance has improved, lift the arm and leg on the same side of the body, with the same breath pattern as above.

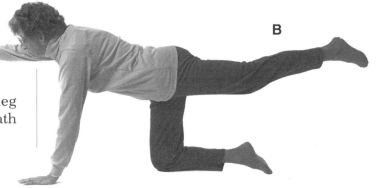

B

BABY POSE

How Will This Exercise Help?

Relieves fatigue. Improves circulation throughout vital organs and brings fresh blood and oxygen to the brain. Improves breathing. Limbers the lower back, hips, knees, and feet. Improves digestion.

Instructors Should Remember . . .

Remind students never to come up quickly from this position—blood draining from the head could cause faintness.

Many students find this position very restful. Encourage them to practice it at home often to remove fatigue.

 Severe hypertension, arthritic knees.

Verbal Instructions

1. **From a hands-and-knees position, be sure the toes are uncurled so that the tops of the feet rest against the floor. Slowly sit back as far as possible.**
   [Ideally, the hips should rest on the heels.]

2. **Bend forward so that your head comes down to the floor in front of your knees. If that position is comfortable, bring your arms down to your sides with the elbows bent so they rest on the floor [A]. Try to relax your whole body so that you go limp — just like a sack of potatoes. Especially relax the back of your neck.**

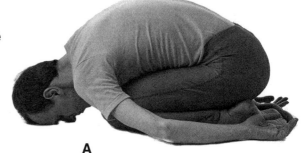

A

3. **Breathe gently and rest.** [Pause 15 to 30 seconds.]

4. **Now slowly come back up to a sitting position. How did that feel?**

Variations

Students who are overweight, or who feel uncomfortable when blood rushes to their head, can rest their head on folded arms in front of their knees.

For students with painful, stiff, or arthritic knees, this exercise can be done across a bed or hassock with a trainer's help [B]. Have the student lie across the bed and reach down to the floor with both hands. Hold the student's shoulders to prevent fear of falling, especially if the student's arms are weak. In this position the head and neck should be relaxed and the position should be held for about a minute, breathing normally. Encourage the student to slide forward so that arms are resting on the floor if possible.

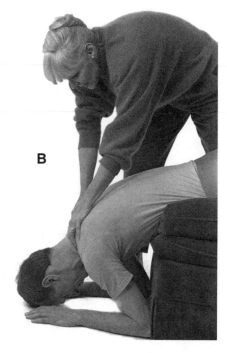

B

INVERTED REST POSE

How Will This Exercise Help?

Tones the entire endocrine system by stimulating thyroid and parathyroid. Improves eyesight, breathing, and circulation. Removes fatigue.

Instructors Should Remember . . .

This exercise should not be done by anyone with high blood pressure, heart disease, or neck problems; substitute the Easy Bridge (page 80) instead. Be sure to stand close to the student while teaching this exercise and be sure the student supports his or her back properly in Step 2. Have students practice on a foam mat or soft carpet to minimize discomfort.

Verbal Instructions

1. Sit on the floor with your knees drawn up to your chest and arms wrapped around your knees. Keep your back rounded and your chin tucked. Now gently roll back and forth a few times, rolling onto your upper back and then forward to a sitting position.

2. Now roll back on your upper back and immediately support your lower back with both hands, resting your elbows on the floor. Keep your knees bent and legs relaxed so your heels are as close to your body as possible. Hold, breathing normally. [Count to five.]

3. Release and gently roll forward to a sitting position, then lie on your back and rest for at least one minute.

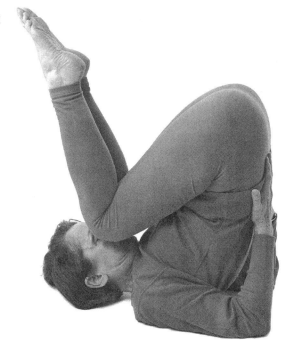

Variations

Students who are afraid to roll back, or who are very stiff, can lie on their back with their hips pressed close to a chair or bed and their legs resting on top of the chair seat or the bed.

INCONTINENCE RELIEF

How Will This Exercise Help?

This special exercise strengthens the groin and abdominal muscles; if done regularly, it can help prevent accidental voiding.

Instructors Should Remember . . .

In this exercise, it is important to expel the air completely in order to achieve the full effect. After tightening the muscles and holding, be sure students release the muscles before breathing in. Encourage students to practice this exercise at home at least twice a day; it can be done conveniently lying in bed just after retiring at night and before getting up in the morning.

Verbal Instructions

1. **Lie flat, with legs bent and feet flat on the bed or floor, separated by several inches. Put your arms at your sides, palms up.** [This position is similar to that for the Easy Bridge except for the hand position: see p. 80.] **Breathe in and out three times through your nose.**

2. **Breathe out through the nose completely, then take a deep breath in. Hold the breath in.** [Count to three.]

3. **Then breathe out as hard as you can until all the breath is gone, forcing the breath out until you are completely empty of breath. You will feel your stomach muscles tighten.**

4. **Now with the breath completely out, suck in all of your stomach, pelvic, and buttock muscles toward your spine as hard as you can. Hold.** [Count to three.]

5. **Release your muscles and breathe in through your nose deeply. Let the breath out normally. Rest a moment.**

   [Repeat for a total of three to five repetitions, resting between each one.]

CHAPTER 6

TEACHING BETTER BREATHING

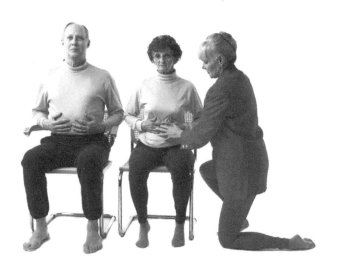

As you've noticed throughout the exercise chapters, each technique includes a specific breath pattern, which is essential for the exercise to be effective. Note also that each technique begins with three complete breaths. Teaching people how to breathe before they start to move brings their attention to the breath, which deepens it.

Older adults, especially if they have become more inactive during their later years, tend to breathe less deeply; this contributes to feelings of lethargy and weakness which, in turn, contributes to further inactivity. Unless muscles are exercised, as they age they lose their elasticity — including the muscles that control respiration, such as the intercostal muscles between the ribs. Poor posture and weak back and stomach muscles create a chronic slouch that also inhibits breathing. The combination of inactivity, slouching, and muscle stiffness combines to create a state of more or less severe oxygen deprivation — and also contributes to depression.

Easy Does It Yoga teaches a complete diaphragmatic breath that trains the lungs to fill and empty more fully, allowing more oxygen in and pushing more waste products out. The practice of breathing deeply throughout the Easy Does It Yoga class session encourages students to practice breathing more deeply at other times of the day as well, and the exercises that strengthen the back and expand the chest wall increase breath capacity by stretching previously unused muscles and improving posture. Increased oxygen to the brain results in a happier, more alert, and more energetic individual who approaches life with more zest.

Breathing and Stress Management

Deep, rhythmic breathing also has the effect of calming and focusing one's attention, and can be used to relieve anxiety, anger, pain, fear, or other strong feelings associated with stress that may be hindering daily functioning. When you teach breathing, talk about the different situations in life that might be stressful, such as family problems, living on a fixed income and other financial concerns, medical or dental problems, loneliness. Discuss how the breath is closely related to emotion: imagine what happens to the breath when you are depressed, angry, or excited. In Easy Does It Yoga, breathing techniques can be used to change one's mood. Encourage students to experiment with changing their breathing in order to help themselves feel better.

Teaching Breathing Techniques

There are several important aspects to learning how to breathe better that should be emphasized often:

Correct posture. Breathing should be taught with the student sitting in a straight chair, sitting away from the chair back. If the student's feet do not rest comfortably on the floor, put a pillow or telephone book under his or her feet. It is easier to maintain a straight back if there is a slight downward slant from hips to knees; create this by tucking the toes under the chair slightly. A straight back can also be reinforced by practicing the Belly Breath against a wall (see illustration). The student is instructed to sit with hips and shoulders touching the wall, which prevents the back from slouching forward during exhalation.

Breathing can also be taught with the student lying flat in bed or on the floor, with knees bent (see Relaxing Breath, page 93). They should not have a pillow under their head, or any pressure on the back of the neck.

Always breathe through the nose. Many people approach any exercise class with the idea of breathing out through pursed lips, as is done in many calisthenic-type exercise programs. In Easy Does It Yoga, all breathing is done through the nose unless the student has a specific airways problem. Breathing through the nose affects the nervous system differently from mouth breathing. It allows for a more deliberate inhalation and exhalation and improves concentration.

Use stomach muscles. To use the diaphragm fully, the belly should go OUT when the breath comes in, and should come IN when the breath goes out. This is opposite to the way most of your students will have been breathing. Most people breathe from the upper portion of their chest; when they breathe in, they suck their stomach in so that the chest expands more. In the breathing techniques taught in this section, your most important task will be to show students how to reverse their usual breathing pattern so they learn to use their diaphragm and belly muscles to breathe as well as their upper chest. We suggest that you work individually with each student, being liberal with your praise at every success. In the Belly Breath, your students will have their hands on their belly to help their breath move in and out correctly. Kneel beside your students and place one hand in the small of their back and the other *over their own hands* on their belly (see illustration). As you instruct students to breathe in and out, you will be able to push in and pull out on their hands to help them experience how their belly should be moving with the breath. At the same time, you can help them keep their back straight with slight support of your other hand at the small of their back. Students will be able to feel their breath in their lower back as well as their stomach.

Wear loose clothing. Students with tight waistbands or girdles will have trouble breathing correctly. Encourage students to wear loose, comfortable, warm clothing to class so they can breathe freely. Long pants are better than shorts, to keep the legs warm.

BELLY BREATH

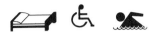

How Will This Exercise Help?

Establishes diaphragmatic breathing pattern, strengthens and more fully uses the diaphragm and surrounding muscles, tones the abdominal muscles. This type of breathing is vital for the most efficient respiration and is best for rehabilitating those with chronic lung disease. In normal older people it improves oxygenation. Slow, deep breathing helps with stress coping, emotional balance, and relaxation.

Instructors Should Remember . . .

Check posture frequently. Help students individually. Start with ten repetitions. Be sure students are breathing in *and* out through the nose.

Verbal Instructions

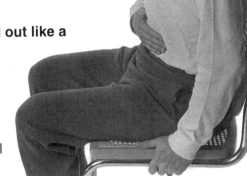

A

1. Sit up straight and away from the back of your chair. Spread your fingers and hands low on your belly.

2. Slowly breathe in deeply through your nose.

3. As you begin to breathe out, push firmly on your belly in and up, gently forcing the air out with your hands [A].

4. As you start to breathe in, let your belly drop down and out like a balloon being filled with air [B].

5. As you breathe out, slowly press in and up again with your hands.

6. Relax. How did that feel?

   [Repeat several times, using the phrase, "Breathe in and fill up with air; breathe out and squeeze the air out." Relax for at least a minute after the last repetition.]

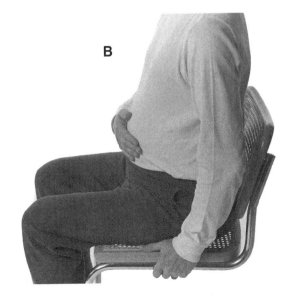

B

Variations

When the Belly Breath is perfected, the sequence can be done without using the hands at all — though use of the hands will help reinforce the correct movement at all times.

Practicing this exercise seated on the steps of a pool will strengthen respiratory muscles due to the increased resistance from the water.

OMPLETE BREATH

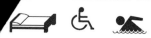

How Will This Exercise Help?

Strengthens and loosens all the respiratory muscles, improves posture, tones abdominal muscles. This exercise is refreshing and invigorating and also has a calming effect. It helps to relieve depression, boredom, and anxiety, and helps to improve self-esteem.

Instructors Should Remember . . .

Remember to check for correct posture throughout the exercise. Students will tend to slouch as they exhale and arch up as they inhale; stress the importance of keeping the head and shoulders steady during the exercise.

The first part of this exercise teaches expansion of the rib cage by raising the arms as the student breathes in. In the second part of the exercise, the hands rest on the hips or legs.

Allow about ten seconds for each breath (five seconds inhalation and five exhalation). In the Complete Breath, the inhalation and exhalation should be roughly equal in length.

Verbal Instructions

1. **Sit up straight, away from the back of your chair, with your arms at your sides.**

2. **Slowly breathe out through your nose, tightening your belly muscles.**

3. **Start to breathe in, belly first, as you raise your arms up in a big circle. Continue breathing in filling your chest and all the way up to your shoulders** [as arms come up over the head].

4. **Now start to breathe out, starting from your shoulders and chest, and lowering your arms to your sides in time with your breath. Pull in your belly to get the last of the air out.**

5. **Relax. How did that feel?**

   [Repeat 5 to 10 times. Rest for at least a minute after the last repetition.]

6. **Now put your hands on your hips or thighs, but keep your arms away from your rib cage so you can breathe deeply.**

7. **Breathe out through your nose, tightening your belly muscles.**

8. **Breathe in, pushing your belly out and filling from the bottom, then expanding your chest.**

9. **Now breathe out, letting your shoulders and chest relax first, then tightening your belly to push the last of the air out.**

   [Repeat several times, making the inhalation and exhalation roughly equal in length.]

Variations

This exercise is also effective done in the pool.

HUMMING BREATH

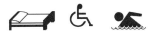

How Will This Exercise Help?

Strengthens breathing muscles by emphasizing inhalation and exhalation. Improves concentration by focusing on a steady sound while exhaling.

Instructors Should Remember . . .

Some students may feel embarrassed at first if their voice is "wobbly" during the humming breath. Do the exercise with your class every time to help them feel more at ease. You can even joke about the fact that "this isn't an audition for the Met!" and that the tunefulness of the sound is not an issue. Encourage a loud, robust tone, and stress the benefits of the exercise: stronger breathing muscles and greater concentration.

Verbal Instructions

1. **Sit straight in your chair with hands on your hips. Breathe in and out three times.**

2. **Breathe in completely a little faster than usual.**

3. **Now breathe out with an audible "hummmm" sound, making the tone steady and loud until your breath is gone. Let the sound vibrate in your throat, and keep pushing with your belly muscles so that the sound doesn't trail off at the end.**

[Demonstrate once, then repeat with the class several times.]

RELAXING BREATH

How Will This Exercise Help?

This breathing exercise can be done by anyone in bed or on the floor. The back is naturally kept straight and the student can concentrate on the movement of the belly and chest during the breath practice. This exercise can help with insomnia.

Instructors Should Remember . . .

Do not let students use a pillow under their head (unless a medical problem requires it) or any pressure on the back of the neck. The legs are most restful if the toes are pointed slightly in, so that the knees rest together. For active students, this is a good way to end a session of floor exercises; you can move directly from the Relaxing Breath to the lying down complete relaxation (see Chapter 7).

Verbal Instructions

1. **Lie on your back with your knees bent. Separate your feet and lean your knees against each other. Place your hands on your belly just as in the Belly Breath. Close your eyes.**

2. **Start to breathe in and out through your nose, just as in the Complete Breath. Your belly will rise up as you inhale and drop down as you exhale. Focus your attention on the sound and feeling of the breath and try to ignore any other sounds or thoughts. Feel yourself relaxing more each time you exhale.**

3. **Continue breathing for about 3 minutes, then relax with eyes closed.**

STOMACH LIFT

How Will This Exercise Help?

Limbers spine, strengthens abdominal and back muscles, improves breathing and digestive function. Helps prevent incontinence.

Instructors Should Remember . . .

Students with painful or arthritic knees should have a foam mat or pillow under their knees; the exercise can also be done on a firm bed. Breathe in and out through the nose.

⊖ Disk problems in the lower back or neck.

Verbal Instructions

1. **Start on your hands and knees. Breathe in and out three times through your nose.**

2. **Breathe out completely, then breathe in as you arch your back and look up toward the ceiling [A].**

3. **Breathe out as you round your back, tuck your chin toward your chest and pull in and up on your stomach muscles [B]. Hold. [Count to three.]**

4. **Breathe in and relax. How did that feel?**

   [Repeat three times.]

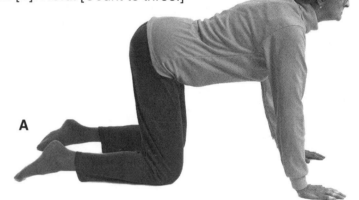

A

Variations

Students who are unable to put weight on their knees can do this exercise standing: Start by separating the feet several inches, bending the knees, and bracing the hands on the knees, keeping the arms straight. Proceed with the exercise as above. Do not allow students to close their eyes because they might lose their balance.

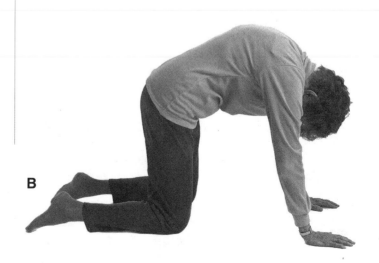

B

CHAPTER 7

TEACHING RELAXATION

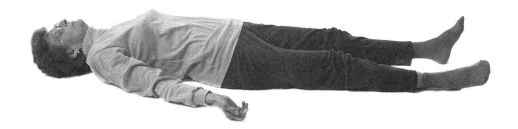

Learning to relax at will is an important component of stress management, and this can only be achieved by practicing a little every day. End every exercise session with 10 to 15 minutes of relaxation, and encourage students to practice this technique every day at home.

THE RELAXATION PROCEDURE

How Will This Exercise Help?

Relaxation teaches students how to become aware of muscle tension so they can relax it before it develops into headaches, back pain, or joint stiffness. Relaxation also gives students a quiet, centered feeling that will help them respond to common life crises without excessive tension and anxiety.

Relaxation makes rest more effective, helps reduce chronic pain complaints, and sharpens the kinesthetic sense (the awareness of where one's body is in space). Many believe that anxiety, irritability, and nervousness are also reduced by less physical tension. Practitioners of regular relaxation also learn to control self-defeating, self-limiting, and frequently unconscious thought patterns, because the habit of quieting one's thoughts during relaxation tends to reinforce positive thoughts while discouraging harmful ones.

Instructors Should Remember . . .

Blood pressure and muscle tone naturally decrease during relaxation; after relaxation, a five-minute period of readjustment is required before resuming normal activities.

Be watchful for patients falling into deep sleep and possibly falling out of their chairs. Students who are taking antipsychotic medication may experience disorientation and should practice relaxation for shorter periods at first; they will also be more comfortable lying down for relaxation

For comfortable posture, the hips should be pressed against the back of the chair so the spine will be comfortably straight without slouching or straining. Separate the legs a few inches and turn the toes inward so that the knees rest together comfortably. It is important for each student to have

95

a sweater or shawl to wrap up in during the relaxation. When one becomes very quiet, body temperature naturally drops slightly, so it is important to stay warm. Also, a wrap provides a psychological feeling of protection while one's eyes are closed and one is in a quiet, vulnerable state.

This technique can also be done lying in bed or on the floor. Students should try not to use a pillow under the head, but pillows under the knees will release any tension in the lower back.

Verbal Instructions

1. **Sit back in your chair and straighten up as much as possible without straining. Put your hands in your lap and close your eyes.** [For lying down version: "Lie comfortably on your back with legs together, arms at your sides, palms up. Close your eyes."]

2. **Now, take three deep breaths, relaxing more and more with each exhalation** [count breaths].

3. **Bring your attention to your face and eyes and feel them relax** [pause].

4. **Let your neck and shoulders relax, and now feel your arms and hands become warm and relaxed, too** [pause].

5. **Take another deep breath, and let go of more tension as you breathe out.**

6. **Feel your heart beating in your chest, and let it relax too** [pause].

7. **Let all your belly muscles relax as you feel them move rhythmically with your breath** [pause].

8. **Feel your legs and feet become empty** [pause], **and relax your back, shoulders, and neck again** [pause].

9. **Relax the inside of your head, even your scalp and brain** [pause].

10. **Now, look again at your forehead, eyes, face, and jaw, and make sure they are relaxed completely** [pause].

11. **Let your breathing relax even more, and feel total relaxation in your upper back, shoulders, and neck** [pause].

12. **Now, for just a few moments, we are going to be completely still, without talking, looking around, or moving even one muscle.**

    [Be quiet and watchful for 30 seconds to 1 minute.]

13. **Now, look inside yourself and see how quiet you have become** [pause]. **And now, I want you to breathe a little deeper.**

14. **Find your hands and gently make fists** [pause], **and now straighten out your legs and point your toes back toward your chin** [pause].

15. **Now, take in a really deep breath. Breathe out, then relax and breathe normally. Make fists; open and close your hands, and flap your feet back and forth. Stretch your arms up toward the ceiling. Open your eyes when you wish.**

    [Spend at least five minutes asking students to talk about their sensations, feelings, and thoughts during the relaxation period, and then encourage the students to begin moving around again, slowly at first, then resuming normal activity levels.]

96

CHAPTER 8

SUGGESTED CURRICULUM OUTLINES

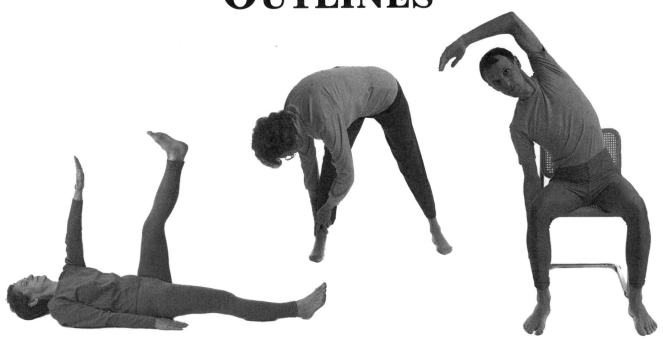

The curriculum you develop for your class — whether the class is composed of several residents in a nursing home or simply your elderly parent at home — should be unique to the physical condition and stamina of your students. When you find out about medical conditions (see Chapter 1) you will be able to outline a class format that will challenge your students without overwhelming them. In this chapter you will find outlines for a 30-minute lecture-demonstration and four-week courses for 1) those in wheelchairs, 2) bedridden students, 3) semi-active students, and 4) active students. Use these as models for how to combine the techniques for varied physical abilities. Note that the sequence of exercises flows from seated to standing to floor, and within each section, exercises are listed from easiest to most difficult (as they are presented in this book). When you add exercises, insert them so your new routine flows smoothly.

Remember to rest frequently — at least after every three or four exercises; more often if students are quite frail. The total time you spend in a class will vary: Frail students will ideally respond best to shorter class times (20-30 minutes) meeting every day; more active students can usually practice in 45- to 60-minute sessions once or twice a week. Each class session is organized roughly as follows:

Warm-up sequence
Breathing techniques
Seated exercises
Standing exercises
Floor exercises
Breathing techniques
Relaxation procedure
(seated in chairs or lying down)
Brief discussion

Remember that one of your goals is to motivate your students to practice Easy Does It Yoga at home on their own. No one feels like practicing something that hurts or that feels too much like work, so make your classes fun, interesting, and stimulating: For instance, bring in newspaper or magazine articles about current health or nutrition issues for discussion, or invite students to bring in a relative or friend to learn with them. We do not recommend the use of music in an Easy Does It Yoga class, as it distracts students from paying attention to their bodies and minds. Frequently repeat the benefits of the techniques, and, as the class progresses, draw out your students so they notice how the techniques are affecting their health and well-being.

Try to be prepared for each class so you don't have to refer constantly to your notes or to the book. Use your knowledge of your students and your own intuition to create your own special Easy Does It Yoga program.

LECTURE-DEMONSTRATION

The purpose of a lecture-demonstration program is to capture the interest of potential students or trainers by giving them a brief and entertaining experience of Easy Does It Yoga. Choose techniques that can safely be done by anyone in your audience and which illustrate how easy and fun the program is to do. Use anecdotes from your personal experience or from previous classes. Ask the audience to participate, and ask them how they feel after doing the techniques.

Five minutes

Start with a brief introduction about what Easy Does It Yoga is and especially what its practical benefits are for your audience. Briefly describe the type of program you are offering.

Five minutes

Teach the Belly Breath to the group. Emphasize how different it is from normal breathing, and how it helps to "clear the cobwebs away."

Ten minutes

Teach a few simple exercises such as the Arm Reach, Shoulder Roll, Seated Leg Lift, and Frog Pose. Have everyone stand up and try the Strut, Standing Reach, and Lazy Knee Bends. Talk about the practical benefits of each exercise and explain that the class will include both easier and more challenging variations so no one has to be worried about being left behind or becoming bored.

Five minutes

Talk the group through a brief relaxation, and talk about the benefits of learning how to relax your muscles and take a break from stress.

Five minutes

Invite your audience to tell you how they feel after doing these few exercises and to ask any questions. If some of your students from a previous or ongoing program are present, invite them to share their experiences or even demonstrate some of the techniques.

WHEELCHAIR ROUTINE

Chairs should be locked in place and feet should be firmly supported. Encourage wheelchair clients to do the Bed Routine exercises every day as well to help prevent sores, improve circulation, and keep joints and muscles from becoming stiff and weak. Some clients may feel insecure about attempting forward-bending exercises, especially if their legs are weak. Stand close to your student and be ready to provide support if needed. Breathing and relaxation training is very important. Encourage students to practice the techniques at other times of the day.

Week 1

Warm-up Sequence, pp. 20–21
Belly Breath, p. 91
Shoulder Roll, p. 26
Elbow Roll, p. 25
Arm Reaches, p. 24
Neck Stretches, pp. 30–31
Arm Circles, p. 28
Rest Sequence, p. 21
Foot Flap and Ankle Rotation, p. 41
Seated Leg Lifts, pp. 40–41
Seated Full Bend Breath, pp. 46–47
Massage, pp. 32–33
Seated Knee Squeeze, p. 42
Frog Pose, p. 37
Relaxation Procedure, pp. 95–96

Week 2, add:

Complete Breath, p. 92
Facial Exercises, p. 34
Throat Tightener, p. 27
Arm Swing, p. 29
Folded Pose, pp. 44–45
Seated Twist, p. 39
Laughing Bicycle, p. 43

Week 3, add:

Lion, p. 36
Elbow to Knee, p. 50
Eye Exercises, p. 35
Humming Breath, p. 93

Week 4, add:

Full Bend Twist, pp. 48–49
Side Stretch, p. 38

BED ROUTINE

Some seated exercises are included in the routine below, since many students will be able to sit up in bed supported by the headboard or wall, or on the edge of the bed with feet on the floor. Also, many of the upper-body exercises can be done lying on one's side, alternating sides so that one arm works at a time. Do not attempt any forward-bending seated exercises unless the feet are firmly on the floor, and always stand close to your student to provide support if needed. Stress the importance of learning the breathing and relaxation techniques and practicing them at various times of day.

Week 1

Warm-up Sequence, pp. 20–21
Belly Breath, p. 91
Shoulder Roll, p. 26
Elbow Roll, p. 25
Arm Reaches, p. 24
Arm Swing, p. 29
Neck Stretches, pp. 30–31
Foot Flap and Ankle Rotation, p. 41
Knee Squeeze, pp. 78–79
Alternate Toe Touch, p. 81
Massage, pp. 32–33
Sun Pose Stretch, p. 73
Easy Bridge, p. 80
Relaxation Procedure, pp. 95–96

Week 2, add:

Facial Exercises, p. 34

Throat Tightener, p. 27
Seated Knee Squeeze, p. 42
Laughing Bicycle, p. 43
Gentle Twist, p. 76
Incontinence Relief, p. 88
Complete Breath, p. 92

Week 3, add:

Lower Back Stretch, p. 82
Back Strengtheners, p. 84
Sun Pose Stretch, p. 73
Humming Breath, p. 93

Week 4, add:

Seated Sun Pose, p. 74
Easy Cobra Lift, p. 83
Easy Bridge, p. 80
Relaxing Breath, p. 93

SEMI-ACTIVE ROUTINE

This routine is suitable for students who are mobile but unable to live independently due to chronic illness, convalescence, or disability. Most exercises are done in chairs or standing holding on to a support, and the technique for getting down on the floor is introduced very gradually. It may take more than four weeks for some students to build the strength needed for floor exercises. Encourage students to try some of the floor exercises in bed at home. Note that in this and the following routine for more active students, groups of chair and standing exercises are alternated to provide a rest.

Week 1

Seated
Warm-up Sequence, pp. 20–21
Belly Breath, p. 91
Shoulder Roll, p. 26
Elbow Roll, p. 25
Arm Reaches, p. 24
Neck Stretches, pp. 30–31
Massage, pp. 32–33

Standing
Standing Reach, p. 56
Standing Leg Lifts, p. 60
Strut, p. 55
Ankle Strengthener, p. 55
Lazy Knee Bends, p. 68
Leg and Arm Strengtheners, p. 69

Seated
Arm Swing, p. 29
Seated Knee Squeeze, p. 42
Seated Twist, p. 39
Seated Leg Lifts, pp. 40–41
Folded Pose, pp. 44–45
Foot Flap and Ankle Rotation, p. 41
Seated Full Bend Breath, pp. 46–47
Belly Breath, p. 91
Relaxation Procedure, pp. 95–96

Week 2, add:

Seated
Complete Breath, p. 92
Arm Circles, p. 28
Throat Tightener, p. 27
Seated Knee Squeeze, p. 42
Full Bend Twist, pp. 48–49

Standing
Tip-Toe Balance, p. 57

Seated
Lion, p. 36

Frog Pose, p. 37
Elbow to Knee, p. 50
Side Stretch, p. 38
Laughing Bicycle, p. 43

Floor
Getting Down on the Floor, pp. 70–72
Sun Pose Stretch, p. 73
Relaxing Breath, p. 93

Week 3, add:

Seated
Humming Breath, p. 93
Facial Exercises, p. 34
Eye Exercises, p. 35
Full Bend Twist, pp. 48–49

Standing
Rear Leg Lifts, p. 64
Rear Arm Lift, p. 54
Gentle Full Bend, pp. 58-59

Floor
Seated Sun Pose, p. 74
Easy Cobra Lift, p. 83
Gentle Twist, p. 76
Incontinence Relief, p. 88
Humming Breath, p. 93

Week 4, add:

Seated
Folded Pose, pp. 44–45

Standing
Tree Pose, p. 63

Floor
Alternate Tortoise Stretch, p. 77
Laughing Bicycle, p. 43
Alternate Toe Touch, p. 81
Easy Bridge, p. 80
Stomach Lift, p. 94

ACTIVE ROUTINE

In this routine, most warm-ups can be done standing. If students are comfortable exercising on the floor, do the relaxation exercise lying down, with pillows under the knees to reduce pressure in the lower back, but no pillow under the head. Some breathing may be done lying down also.

Week 1

Standing
Warm-up Sequence, pp. 20–21
Shoulder Roll, p. 26
Elbow Roll, p. 25
Arm Reaches, p. 24
Neck Stretches, pp. 30–31
Arm Circles, p. 28

Seated
Arm Swing, p. 29
Elbow to Knee, p. 50
Seated Leg Lifts, pp. 40–41
Seated Knee Squeeze, p. 42
Massage, pp. 32–33
Lion, p. 36
Seated Full Bend Breath, pp. 46–47
Seated Twist, p. 39

Standing
Standing Reach, p. 56
Strut, p. 55
Standing Leg Lifts, p. 60
Tree Pose, p. 63
Gentle Full Bends, pp. 58–59

Floor
Getting Down on the Floor, pp. 70–72
Foot Flaps and Ankle Rotation, p. 41
Sun Pose Stretch, p. 73
Gentle Twist, p. 76
Knee Squeeze, pp. 78-79

Seated
Belly Breath, p. 91
Complete Breath, p. 92
Relaxation Procedure, pp. 95–96

Week 2, add:

Seated
Throat Tightener, p. 27
Full Bend Twist, pp. 48–49
Folded Pose, pp. 44–45
Frog Pose, p. 37

Standing
Tip-Toe Balance, p. 57
Rear Leg Lifts, p. 64
Super Balance Pose, p. 65
Rear Arm Lift, p. 54

Seated
Side Stretch, p. 38
Elbow to Knee, p. 50

Floor
Back Strengtheners, p. 84
Easy Bridge, p. 80
Incontinence Relief, p. 88
Alternate Toe Touch, p. 81
Easy Cobra Lift, p. 83
Laughing Bicycle, p. 43
Stomach Lift, p. 94

Week 3, add:

Seated
Facial Exercises, p. 34

Standing
Standing Knee Squeeze, p. 61
Simple Alternate Triangle, p. 62

Seated
Shoulder to Knee, p. 51
Eye Exercises, p. 35
Lion, p. 36
Humming Breath, p. 93

Floor
Lower Back Stretch, p. 82
Back Strengtheners, p. 84
Easy Cobra Lift, p. 83
Baby Pose, p. 86

Week 4, add:
Super Balance Pose, p. 65
Simple Alternate Triangle, p. 66
Seated Leg Lifts, pp. 40–41
Alternate Tortoise Stretch, p. 77
All Fours Lift, p. 85
Inverted Rest Pose, p. 87

Appendix A

Techniques Grouped By Benefit

Face, Neck, Shoulders, Upper Back

Chair

Arm Reaches, p. 24
Shoulder Roll, p. 26
Throat Tightener, p. 27
Arm Swing, p. 29
Elbow Roll, p. 25
Arm Circles, p. 28
Neck Stretches, pp. 30–31
Neck and Shoulder Massage, pp. 32–33
Facial Exercises, p. 34
Eye Exercises, p. 35
Lion, p. 36
Frog Pose, p. 37
Full Bend Twist, pp. 48–49

Standing

Rear Arm Lift, p. 54
Standing Reach, p. 56
Gentle Full Bend, pp. 58–59
Leg and Arm Strengtheners, p. 69

Spinal Flexibility and Strength

Chair

Side Stretch, p. 38
Seated Twist, p. 39
Seated Full Bend Breath, pp. 46–47
Full Bend Twist, p. 48–49
Folded Pose, pp. 44–45
Seated Knee Squeeze, p. 42

Elbow to Knee, p. 50
Shoulder to Knee, p. 51
Frog Pose, p. 37

Standing

Standing Reach, p. 56
Gentle Full Bend, pp. 58–59
Simple Alternate Triangle, p. 62

Floor

Stomach Lift, p. 94
Easy Cobra Lift, p. 83
Back Strengtheners, p. 84
Sun Pose Stretch, p. 73
Seated Sun Pose, p. 74
All Fours Lift, p. 85
Knee Squeeze, pp. 78–79
Easy Alternate Sun Pose, p. 75
Gentle Twist, p. 76
Easy Bridge, p. 80

Strengthening Hips, Legs, Ankles, and Feet

Chair

Seated Knee Squeeze, p. 42
Foot Flaps and Ankle Rotations, p. 41
Side Stretch, p. 38
Seated Sun Pose, p. 74
Seated Leg Lifts, pp. 40–41

Standing

Standing Reach, p. 56
Strut, p. 55
Ankle Strengthener, p. 55

Simple Alternate Triangle, p. 62
Tip–Toe Balance, p. 57
Lazy Knee Bend, p. 68
Rear Leg Lift, p. 64
Super Balance Pose, p. 65
Tree Pose, p. 63
Standing Leg Lifts, p. 60
Standing Knee Squeeze, p. 61
Leg and Arm Strengtheners, p. 69

Floor

All Fours Lift, p. 85
Easy Bridge, p. 80
Easy Alternate Sun Pose, p. 75
Alternate Tortoise Stretch, p. 77
Alternate Toe Touch, p. 81
Lower Back Stretch, p. 82

IMPROVED BREATHING

Chair

Belly Breath, p. 91
Complete Breath, p. 92
Humming Breath, p. 93
Laughing Bicycle, p. 43
Frog Pose, p. 37
Arm Reach, p. 24
Elbow Roll, p. 25
Arm Swing, p. 29
Side Stretch, p. 38
Full Bend Twist, pp. 48–49

Standing

Tip–Toe Balance, p. 57
Rear Arm Lift, p. 54
Standing Reach, p. 56
Gentle Full Bend, p. 58–59

Floor

Easy Cobra Lift, p. 83
Baby Pose, p. 86
Knee Squeeze, pp. 78–79

IMPROVED DIGESTION

Chair

Seated Knee Squeeze, p. 42
Folded Pose, pp. 44–45
Elbow to Knee, p. 50

Shoulder to Knee, p. 51
Seated Twist, p. 39
Seated Full Bend Breath, pp. 46–47
Full Bend Twist, pp. 48–49

Standing

Gentle Full Bend, pp. 58–59
Standing Knee Squeeze, p. 61

Floor

Knee Squeeze, pp. 78–79
Sun Pose Stretch, p. 73
Seated Sun Pose, p. 74
Gentle Twist, p. 76
Stomach Lift, p. 94

ENERGIZERS

Energizers are any techniques that improve oxygenation by expanding the chest wall, increase upper body circulation, bring a fresh blood supply to the head, and/or stretch and contract postural muscles. Examples:

Elbow Roll, p. 25
Shoulder Roll, p. 26
Frog Pose, p. 37
Folded Pose, pp. 44–45
Gentle Full Bends, pp. 58–59
Arm Reaches, p. 24
Laughing Bicycle, p. 43
Arm Swing, p. 29

RELAXERS

Relaxers are any techniques that release tension in the stomach and breathing muscles, release facial tension, compress the abdomen, and/or focus attention inward on the breath process or on the relaxation process. Examples:

Belly Breath, p. 91
Seated Twist, p. 39
Seated Knee Squeeze, p. 42
Humming Breath, p. 93
Lion, p. 36
Facial Exercises, p. 34
Full Bend Twist, pp. 48–49
Folded Pose, pp. 44–45
Easy Cobra Lift, p. 83
Relaxation, pp. 95–96

Appendix B

Additional Resources

Some instructional materials that you might find helpful are available from the American Yoga Association as well as many bookstores and video outlets. To request a catalog, or for information on quantity discounts for trainers, please write or call either center:

American Yoga Association
513 South Orange Avenue
Sarasota, Florida 34236
(813) 953-5859
(800) 226-5859

American Yoga Association
P.O. Box 18105
Cleveland Heights, Ohio 44118
(216) 371-0078

Books

Easy Does It Yoga for Older People. A student's manual. For those with physical limitations, this book includes instruction in specially adapted Yoga exercises which can be done in a chair or in bed, breathing techniques, and meditation. 112 pages. Fully illustrated.

The American Yoga Association Beginner's Manual. Complete instructions for over 90 Yoga exercises and breathing techniques; three 10-week curriculum outlines, and chapters on nutrition, philosophy, stress management, and more. 206 pages. Over 300 photos. (Simon & Schuster, 1987)

20-Minute Yoga Workouts. A series of 20-minute routines including exercise, breathing, and meditation for busy people. Includes "the 20-minute challenge," the 20-minute routine for when you're not at home, sports workouts, and routines for physical limitations. 176 pages. Over 150 photos. (Ballantine, 1995)

Meditation. A collection of excerpts from lectures and classes by Alice Christensen on the subject of meditation, including a section of questions and answers from students. (American Yoga Association, 1994)

Reflections of Love. A collection of excerpts from Alice Christensen's lectures and classes on the subject of love. (American Yoga Association, 1995)

The American Yoga Association Wellness Book. How to relax your mind and body and use special Yoga routines to relieve common health problems such as anxiety, arthritis, hypertension, insomnia, headaches, PMS or menopause, and back and neck pain.

The Light of Yoga. A chronicle of the unusual circumstances that catapulted Alice Christensen into Yoga practice in the early 1950s, including the teachers and experiences that shaped her first years of study.

The Joy of Celibacy. This booklet examines how the unconscious is influenced by the sexual sell of modern advertising and suggests a five-minute celibacy break to help build awareness and self-knowledge.

Conversations with Swami Lakshmanjoo, Volume I: Aspects of Kashmir Shaivism. Edited transcripts of Alice Christensen's interviews with Swami Lakshmanjoo, a great master of Kashmir Shaivism, talking about his childhood and early years in Yoga, plus some basic concepts in the philosophy of Kashmir Shaivism.

Conversations with Swami Lakshmanjoo, Volume II: The Yamas and Niyamas of Patanjali. Edited transcripts of Alice Christensen's dialogues with Swami Lakshmanjoo about these essential ethical guidelines in Yoga.

AUDIOTAPES

Complete Relaxation and Meditation with Alice Christensen. A two-tape audiocassette program that features three guided meditation sessions of varying lengths, including instruction in a seated posture, plus a discussion of meditation experiences.

The "I Love You" Meditation Technique. A 40-minute guided visualization, breathing, and relaxation technique that results in greater self-esteem, confidence, and self-empowerment.

VIDEOTAPES

Basic Yoga. A complete introduction to Yoga that includes exercise, breathing, and relaxation and meditation techniques. Provides detailed instruction in all the techniques including variations for more or less flexibility. Features a 30-minute practice session in a Yoga class setting for a convenient routine to do daily.

Conversations with Swami Lakshmanjoo. A set of three videotapes in which Alice Christensen introduces Swami Lakshmanjoo and talks with him about his background, the philosophy of Kashmir Shaivism, and other topics in Yoga. (Some material corresponds to Volume I of the book *Aspects of Kashmir Shaivism* described above.)

EASY DOES IT YOGA TRAINING PROGRAMS

The American Yoga Association occasionally offers training programs in Easy Does It Yoga. We would also be happy to send a teacher or lecturer to your area for a special training program or lecture on Easy Does It Yoga. We offer a one-day seminar that does not certify you as a Yoga teacher, but it introduces you to the basic concepts of Easy Does It Yoga and provides some hands-on experience in leading another person through the techniques. We also offer a more intensive eight-week course (16 hours, total) for trainers. We would be happy to keep your name on file to be notified about upcoming training programs.

Please write or call either of our two centers for more information.

SUMMARY OF EASY DOES IT YOGA PROGRAM RESEARCH

Easy Does It Yoga (EDY) is a program that consists of specially adapted Yoga exercises for older people — most of which are done in chairs — combined with breathing techniques and relaxation training. All of the techniques are safe and gentle, with endless variations possible according to each individual's physical limitations. Easy Does It Yoga includes sections for exercises that can be done in bed, in a wheelchair, or the pool.

Researchers of the EDY program in the past 20 years have included:

Durand F. Jacobs, Ph.D., Veterans Administration Medical Center, Loma Linda, California.

Roger N. Hess, Ph.D, Douglas Schultz, Ph.D, and Robert W. Scott, M.D., with the support of a matching grant by the Cleveland Foundation and the American Yoga Association.

David Haber, Ph.D., formerly of the University of South Florida, Tampa, supported by an Administration on Aging Title IV-B research grant and the Older Americans Act, Title III.

Research on the EDY program by the Veterans Administration Medical Center showed strong evidence that simple Yoga techniques can reduce somatic and psychological complaints. Participants being evaluated reported improvements in several areas. Our students found a marked reduction in problems resulting from an unhealthy musculoskeletal system, such as pain in the back, arms, and legs, as well as cramps. In addition, students

noticed a general improvement in the functioning of the respiratory system, with less running or bleeding noses, or constant coughing. Many students experienced having an overall improvement of the nervous system. They reported fewer problems of numbness and tingling in the arms and legs, fewer severe headaches, reduced dizziness, and less twitching in the face, head, and shoulder area. Students involved in the program also experienced positive emotional changes. There were large reductions in anxiety symptoms such as nervousness, being easily irritated, and impulsive behavior. Self-esteem increased, and some older students have also reported a renewed interest in sex.

The Cleveland Foundation study explored the effectiveness of the EDY program in augmenting traditional hypertension treatments. Seventy people over the age of 55 who suffered mild to moderate hypertension participated in the project. Half of the participants were assigned to the EDY program, and half to a traditional exercise-to-music program. Both groups met twice weekly for 12 weeks. Clinical status was determined before and after the 12 weeks, and was continued for an additional 12-week follow-up period. Both the EDY program and exercise-to-music program led to reductions in blood pressure, with the Yoga program participants experiencing a statistically significant change. Both groups lost some weight, though neither was significant. As for pulse, both groups reduced pulse rate significantly over the entire 24-week period. A 29-item symptoms checklist included anxiety, depression, tiredness, nervousness, trouble sleeping, stiff joints, and muscle weakness. Results of the symptoms checklist for every comparison in the two groups showed improvement among the Yoga students, which was sustained over the follow-up period. For the controls, although all of the comparisons showed some improvement, only two of the differences were significant, and both of them appeared only at the end of the follow-up period. In summary, both programs led to an improvement in physical well-being, but the features of the Yoga training resulted in a greater feeling of general well-being.

Two senior centers in west central Florida were chosen for an exploratory study, supported by the Administration on Aging, to evaluate the use of Yoga as a preventative health care program. The study was community based, using white volunteers at the SS Center, and black volunteers at the JJ Center. At each site older persons were equally distributed between a Yoga class and a control activity, such as a film series or an art class. Classes were held once a week for 10 weeks at a community site, with daily homework assignments by the students on their own at home. Compared to other group programs with minority elders, drop-out rates were quite low. Yoga participants reduced their systolic blood pressure level in comparison to control persons at the SS Center at the .09 level of significance. Yoga participants at the JJ Center did not lower blood pressure levels in comparison to control persons. Among SS Yoga participants, self-assessed health status improved, as did psychological well-being, in comparison to the control group. At the JJ Center, Yoga participants did not improve on the self-assessed health status measurement or the psychological well-being scale in comparison to the control group. Though equivalent procedures were implemented at both centers, black older students were unable to be motivated to practice Yoga on their own at home. While older students at both centers attended the weekly class on a regular basis, the SS participants practiced Yoga an additional five times per week on average, while the JJ participants practiced only one additional time per week on average. It was concluded that the psychological response to Yoga in the black community may need to improve before we can determine the potential benefits of Yoga with high blood pressure or hypertension. One future direction for low-income, minority elders is to increase class contact from one to three or four times a week. Some analysts believe that more frequent, direct leadership with minority elders is necessary to encourage them to intervene on their own behalf.

The Older Americans Act (Title III) provided funding for a recreation-fitness program for older rural and urban residents of Florida's Tampa Bay Area. Over 100 people, divided into two groups, participated in independent, controlled studies of the impact of Easy Does It Yoga on physical and emotional health. Group I consisted of predominantly white, middle-class female high school graduates living with their spouses, and Group II was nearly one-half black, predominantly female, middle to lower class, junior high school graduates. Within each group about half the participants were randomly assigned to the EDY treatment group, and the other half to the control group. A battery of tests was given to assess the frequency of somatic and nonsomatic complaints (Hopkins Symptom Checklist), to ascertain present levels of tension and nervousness (Spielberger's State Trait Anxiety Inventory), to ascertain present feelings of self-worth (Rosenberg's Self-Esteem Scale), to measure opinions about feelings of accomplishment (Neugarten's Life Satisfaction Index), and to monitor blood pressure. Additional demographic and health care behavior variables were measured. Also, measurements were recorded for the average number of minutes per day and days per week that the Yoga techniques were performed at home. The results of Group I test battery scores showed that the EDY group out-performed the control group on every measure except the somatic and nonsomatic complaints. As well, all changes in mean scores for the EDY group were in a positive direction, except for the life satisfaction score. However, the indicated decrease in life satisfaction was 50% greater for the control group. Test scores for Group II showed that the EDY group did better on every measure compared to the control group. Group I participants practicing the EDY regimen of exercise, breathing, relaxation and meditation techniques at home reported practicing an average of 35 minutes per day. In Group II, EDY participants practiced an average of 32 minutes per day.

INDEX

Technique instructions are indicated by **boldface.**

About the Author

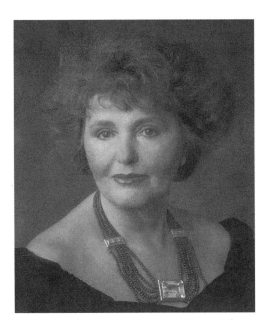

Alice Christensen stands out as a Yoga teacher with the rare ability to make the often-complex ideas and techniques of Yoga accessible to our Western outlook and lifestyle. She established the American Yoga Association (then called the Light of Yoga Society) in 1968, at that time the first and only nonprofit organization in the United States dedicated to education in Yoga, and launched the Easy Does It Yoga program in the late 1960s. Since then, she has supervised many programs in research, direct service, and teacher training that have reached thousands of older adults all over the country. Her emphasis on safety, effectiveness, and enjoyment stands out as an example of the practical approach to Yoga techniques that is the hallmark of her leadership of the American Yoga Association and which has drawn praise from government, health, and research institutions nationwide.

She says: "The Easy Does It Yoga program has been a joy for me to design and implement, primarily because of the enthusiasm of my students. I've seen their faces light up with excitement as they explain to me how Easy Does It Yoga has changed their lives to a positive, independent growth and strength. This has been an unforgettable experience for me."

ABOUT THE AMERICAN YOGA ASSOCIATION

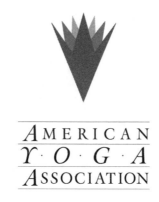

When first founded by Alice Christensen in 1969 as the Light of Yoga Society, the American Yoga Association was the first and only nonprofit, educational organization dedicated to the instruction of classical Yoga in this country. Today, we continue to teach a comprehensive and balanced program of Yoga. Rather than stressing physical culture for its own sake, our core curriculum acknowledges the deeper possibilities of Yoga by teaching meditation and by encouraging the inner-directed awareness that eventually leads to greater self-knowledge. Special programs such as Easy Does It Yoga bring many of the valuable benefits of Yoga to those who may not otherwise be inclined to attempt Yoga practice.

In keeping with our goal of offering the highest quality Yoga instruction possible, we offer regularly scheduled classes and seminars in our centers, in addition to an ever-growing line of instructional books and tapes for home study. There are two American Yoga Association centers in the United States, serving the greater Cleveland and Sarasota/Tampa Bay areas.